UNSTOPPABLE

UNSTOPPABLE

4 STEPS TO TRANSFORM YOUR LIFE

DAVID HAUSER

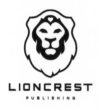

LIONCREST
PUBLISHING

UNSTOPPABLE
4 Steps to Transform Your Life

ISBN   978-1-5445-0324-0 *Hardcover*
       978-1-5445-0325-7 *Paperback*
       978-1-5445-0326-4 *Ebook*
       978-1-5445-0327-1 *Audiobook*

CONTENTS

INTRODUCTION

It was never my dream to write a self-help book about health and wellness. But after almost fifteen years of struggling with my weight and nutrition, it became my imperative.

You see, much like millions of people around the world, I've tried dozens of diets in my lifetime. I've exercised myself to the brink of insanity at the gym. I've even endured five years of relentless endurance sports competitions, which nearly destroyed my knees, yet left me restless inside. All in the name of having control over my weight, how I looked, but most importantly, how I felt.

But none of those things ever delivered the satisfaction and peace of mind I sought. Instead of making me stronger—making me unstoppable—they left me more confused than ever before. I wondered if I was doomed to spend the rest of my life searching for the best diet, the best workout, or the best version of myself. Little did I know the information I was looking for wasn't something that I'd find in popular media about health and wellness. It was something that I'd literally have to find in myself and after years of experimentation, testing, and tracking.

I learned a lot of things from this process. But no lesson was more important than this one: I needed to share this framework with the people out there who are as confused as I was about what it takes to get and stay healthy. For the people who want to make the most of their time with family and friends, and optimize their health at the same time.

Believe me, no one's more surprised than I am to have authored a book that openly acknowledges the shame and guilt I felt when I was overweight in my twenties, as well as my love of yoga. If you'd told me I'd be doing any of this in my early days as an entrepreneur, I would've said you were insane. But the greatest challenges of our lives have the potential to throw open the door to learning. And, although my journey to health and wellness was born of anger and frustration, it has culminated in making me more knowledgeable, more understanding and accepting, and most importantly, more joyful. To me, this is what it means to be unstoppable.

As you may have figured out by now, this isn't your typical book on the topic of health, wellness, or nutrition. Honestly, I couldn't have ever written anything *typical*—after all, I'm a nerd with OCD who grew up programming for fun. But that's what makes this book ideal for the millions of people who have tried the diets and quick fixes and are ready for an actual solution. All that's required on your part is ownership and commitment. You'll have to become your biggest advocate. You'll have to get curious about your own body, conduct experiments, learn from those experiments, and evolve in a way that's unique to *you*. I'll go deeper into what all of this means in the book. And don't worry, it might sound foreign now, but the framework is actually quite simple, and I'll be there to help with the right information along the way. Once you take ownership, the ironic thing is that the Unstoppable Lifestyle will be easier than anything you've ever tried. As was the case in my journey, with the right tools and practices, the path seems to light up in front of you.

And that's not to say you won't face challenges—one of the most significant challenges is from our own culture's entrenched beliefs about health and wellness. But by becoming curious and doing your own research, you'll learn the origin of these beliefs and train a critical lens on the interplay between big business and nutrition. And by using that information to guide experiments, gather data, and interpret results, you'll learn what it means to become truly unstoppable.

Let your journey truly begin now!

PART I

MY STORY

CHAPTER 1

THE JOURNEY

Whether you realize it or not, you embark on a health and wellness journey with each new day. From the moment you open your eyes in the morning until you go to sleep at night, you're making decisions that have the potential to positively or negatively impact your quality of life. That's why what you eat, drink, and think, as well as how you move your body (or not) plays a pivotal role in your journey to health and wellness. Make the right decisions about these things consistently, and more than likely, you'll lead a healthy life. Make the wrong ones and you could suffer serious setbacks on your journey.

Now, I'm not saying all of this to scare you.

On the contrary, actually: I say this to empower you. That's because the right decisions have the potential to serve as entry points into the lives we want to lead, the way we want our bodies to look, and how we want to feel.

But here's the thing: being healthy is hard work. It means making the right decisions from the time we wake up until we go to sleep at night. Being sick, on the other hand—well, that's *easy*. It requires no change in behavior and eliminates the need to make the right decisions all the time about the food you eat or how you treat your body. You can do as you please and take advantage of all that life has to offer.

That is, until you physically can't.

As someone who has struggled with diet, exercise, and health for most of my life, I can attest: being sick was incredibly easy—at first. But over time, being sick held me back from truly taking advantage of all that life has to offer. The decisions I made about what I put in my body and how I moved it started to have massively negative consequences. When my body started to shut down, that's when I started to view decision-making differently.

Instead of obstacles to my happiness, I started to view decisions as small units of potential change—units that, when broken down, could be optimized.

Here's a quick, if oversimplified, example: when confronted with the right food or the wrong food for my body, I could make the decision to go with the food that would give me energy and clear my mind, or I could go with the lesser option. When I changed the way I viewed decision-making, I started to look at scenarios like this one as moments to optimize life starting on a much smaller scale. But when added up, I discovered that all those smaller optimizations translated into tremendous gains in health and wellness.

Makes sense, right? I think so.

But, strangely, our performance-driven and success-obsessed culture tends to overlook this approach to health and wellness. Few people have considered what it means to optimize their time, energy, and resources to lead richer, fuller, healthier lives simply by optimizing their decision-making process. Though every individual is on their own health journey simply by being alive, many haven't been intentional about choosing their *destination*. As an entrepreneur over the last fifteen years, I've seen very ambitious, professionally-minded individuals go about making optimizations in their businesses, in their schedules, and for their employees, but completely overlook making optimizations to body and mind. This has always surprised me, but it also makes clear how even the most driven among us don't think about optimizing things like sleep, exercise, and diet the way we do many other things in our lives.

Instead, I've found that most people who are interested in embarking on their own health and wellness journey are guided by myths that emerge from the pseudoscientific information popularized in the media. As a result, many people think health revolves around counting calories and steps, doing daily cardio exercise, lowering cholesterol, eating low-fat foods, and the like. Though common, accepting this information as truth is dangerous in many ways. That's because much of this information is rooted in faulty science, or shared by brands or spokespeople that have been paid to endorse products. When these products and methodologies don't work as promised, they're understandably frustrated and disappointed.

This reflects my journey to health and wellness, too.

Throughout my twenties and early thirties, I believed in the popular health narratives that seemed to come and go with each passing year:

Burn more calories than you take in and you'll lose weight.

Avoid high-fat foods and you'll keep cholesterol in a healthy range.

Do cardio every day.

These are just some of the health mantras I repeated to

myself while I struggled with my weight, and they dictated my approach to fitness and health. If I felt low on energy, I vowed to do more cardio. When my doctor said my cholesterol was high, I eliminated fatty foods from my diet. But none of it worked. The symptoms always continued, no matter how strict I was with myself. Frustratingly, during this time, popular pseudoscience provided zero answers for why I felt the way I did.

And that's why I decided to write this book—to give people who are searching for answers some place to start. To give people a no-bullshit alternative to the empty health information that's everywhere these days. I also wrote this book because when I set out on my own journey, I wish I'd had a resource like this to parse fact from fiction when it comes to health and wellness, and to help me reach my personal goals.

Once I decided to take matters into my own hands, I started to question everything I'd been led to believe was true about diet, health, medicine, and more. I spent ridiculous amounts of time, money, and energy exploring those areas in an effort to optimize my own life, body, and mind.

The end result?

This book.

Not only will it save you time, money, and energy, as well as help you to jumpstart your journey, but it'll serve as a shortcut for finding the right strategies for optimizing your life and becoming unstoppable. It'll also help you to achieve your own "magic moments"—the name I gave to those times when you really start to see the sum of good decision-making in everyday life. For me, those magical moments were things like losing and *keeping* weight off, finally feeling comfortable taking my shirt off in yoga, and not feeling hungry all the time.

Before we go any further, one thing I want you to know: I understand how hard this is. Over the years, I've felt insecure, self-conscious, and ashamed of my own shortcomings. I've felt like I wasn't doing enough, not limiting myself enough, and it put me in a bad place. I know it can be tough to imagine how to get from where you are today to where you want to be tomorrow. But I'm here to tell you that change is possible if you enter into this journey with your eyes wide open, and with real intention. After all, you only have one life, one body, and one mind. Imagine what it would look like to make the most of them?

Computer scientist Alan Keys probably said it best: "Our ability to open the future will depend not on how well we learn but how well we are able to unlearn." I invite you on this journey with the caveat that it'll require a lot of *unlearning* of thinking and behaviors that feel familiar and "right." It'll be hard. But, in the end, the framework, the practices, and the commitment will make you truly unstoppable.

Let's go.

CHAPTER 2

RECURRING FRUSTRATIONS

There are two dark clouds that have always hovered over me: one, I've always felt fat; and two, I've always felt hungry.

These two deep-seated notions have often made me feel as if I was scrambling aimlessly as I tested different diets and exercise fads. No matter how strict I was in following a new diet or exercise, those two dark clouds remained. Over time, I struggled to manage these feelings. Because I always felt fat, I didn't feel like I should eat. But if I didn't eat, I never had any energy. It was a terrible cycle.

Maybe your struggles are similar, maybe not. Maybe you, like me, have judged yourself as you look in the mirror or work out next to someone at the gym. And maybe this judgment has led you to try all kinds of different diets or dedicate yourself to new workouts. No matter your struggle, the truth is that just about everyone I know is self-conscious about something. Most have aching insecurities. Most people are way too hard on themselves. Most judge themselves harshly for their lives, bodies, and the choices they make that involve them. But right now, let's transform these areas into opportunities for optimization instead of judgment.

THE CRUX OF THE PROBLEM

My own journey, like many, began with trying to get my weight under control. This began in college. In high school, though I was aware of being overweight, I didn't care so much about it. I ate until I felt full. Actually, because I ate so quickly, the truth is that I often ate *beyond* being full. But this didn't take a serious toll on me since I was growing taller with each passing month. I actually thought I was quite healthy in high school because I was cooking my own meals—unlike many high school students—and playing sports. Plus, I could hide my body fat in the mandatory suit coats that we had to wear each day at prep school, or beneath my football uniform on the field. If I didn't see it, I thought, it wasn't there.

When I got to college, I could no longer hide in a uniform.

I struggled because, for the first time, I had to actually think about what I wore each day. In freshman year, I had an unlimited meal plan and a cafeteria a few steps from my dorm, which didn't help matters. I quickly gained the freshman fifteen at the very same time I was navigating the experience of living in a co-ed dorm on campus. For the first time in my life, I felt shame when I looked at myself in the mirror.

Naturally, I wanted to fix this problem. So I did my research, absorbed the advice of friends, and so-called experts in the media, and decided I needed to do cardio—every single day. One thing to know about me: I'm a man of commitment and routine. So I *dedicated* myself to going to the gym every morning, and never missed a day. I remember at one point I ran regularly on the elliptical at the university gym each day for six weeks straight.

One big problem, though.

I didn't lose any weight.

This confused me. After all, I was working out more than I'd ever worked out before and was burning lots of calories.

Amidst this frustration and wondering what else I needed to do, I started to more closely evaluate my food consumption. Since gaining the "freshman fifteen," I'd moved off campus and had started eating less in the school cafeteria. But as a typical college kid, I was still eating all kinds of junk in my apartment—things like ramen noodles and macaroni and cheese. Anxious to see results, I cut back on those foods and tried meal replacement shakes from the then-popular SlimFast brand. Though they were expensive, I was determined to lose weight, so I fully committed to the SlimFast diet. I would eat a shake for breakfast, a shake for lunch, and then I would go to the cafeteria for dinner for my first "real" meal of the day, where I'd be sure to only consume low-fat foods (which, by the way, included low-fat desserts). Much to my surprise, this "diet" seemed to work. I lost about ten pounds in sixty days, chipping away at the weight I added my freshman year.

The problem was that the meal replacement approach was impossible to continue long-term. As a college kid, I couldn't afford to keep buying a steady supply of Slim-Fast shakes to consume twice a day. My weight also plateaued after losing ten pounds. And, most importantly, it didn't work physically because I was absolutely *miserable* on this routine. I was constantly hungry and spent each day thinking about food. This was especially problematic because, at the time, I not only was a full-time student, but I'd just launched a software-as-a-service company called Grasshopper. With a new company that was growing rapidly, not having energy just wasn't an option. Hunger made me sleepy and caused brain fog. But I also had a short temper and no idea why. In short, I was incredibly unhealthy.

But I did learn something from the SlimFast experiment: food mattered. And, if I wanted to lose weight, I needed to do more than simply go to the gym and run on the elliptical seven days a week like a maniac. So, in deciding to eat more than one meal and two shakes a day, I focused on making sure that my meals aligned with the general consensus for nutrition at the time: low fat, high carb, and no red meat. I was still eating processed foods, but I figured if a bag of chips or popcorn said that it was low-fat, then it had to be healthy.

At that time, I also began calorie counting. So, even if I splurged one night and ordered a pizza because I needed the energy to pull an all-nighter, I then made up for it the next day at the gym and would run on the elliptical for 90 to 120 minutes to try and burn the calories I consumed the night before. In exchange for the occasional caloric splurge, I'd sometimes spend two hours on the elliptical burning off the late-night takeout. For a while, calorie counting was a security blanket: it allowed me to eat whatever I wanted to eat as long as I was willing to burn those calories at the gym.

I felt better for a while with this routine. I also had more energy calorie counting than when I was doing the Slim-Fast approach. But slowly, I began gaining all the weight back. When I gained back all the weight I'd lost, I immediately went back to the SlimFast. I was miserable, but it was a short-term solution to what was clearly a long-term problem for me.

At the time I couldn't help but wonder: was this just the way it was going to be? Never losing more than ten pounds and being miserable while doing so?

No matter how hard I tried, it felt like I would always be both fat and hungry. And whenever I didn't get the results I was looking for, I felt like it was all my fault for not succeeding—for breaking down and eating a pizza late, or not burning enough calories at the gym. My reaction every time I stepped onto the scale was, "I'm not doing enough."

And so, the cycle continued as follows: I'd work out more, then feel hungrier. When I gave myself the food I craved, I'd feel guilty for eating. This cycle was incredibly maddening, but it continued for the next several years.

HEALTH AND BUSINESS

I've always been a hard worker. I've had to be. I was diagnosed with a learning disability at an early age and had to be tutored extensively throughout elementary and middle school just to get by academically. Reading was extremely difficult for me, and whenever we read passages from books aloud in English class, my heart would start to race because I was so nervous I'd get called on to read in front of my friends. These insecurities, however, never made me cave to feelings of inadequacy. Instead, they helped me to understand my unique learning style. What's more, they fueled my drive to find other areas to excel in and prove people wrong. Today, I realize this experience made me successful in life. I now consider this disability to be my greatest gift in life because I learned how to learn.

One of the areas in which I was determined to excel was entrepreneurship and business. I guess you could say that entrepreneurship has always been in my blood. In middle school, I made jewelry and sold it. When I was a junior in high school, I read about an affiliate marketing company based out of New York City that intrigued me, so I simply called up the owner, a Harvard Business School graduate, and bluntly told him that I wanted to work for him. He told me to come by the office, and, though he was probably shocked to discover that I was so young, we ended up starting a company together, which is still around today. After that, I attended Babson College in Massachusetts. In my sophomore year, I built and launched Grasshopper, a virtual phone system for entrepreneurs. Honestly, it was shitty software at the time, but because we were tapping into a massive void in the small business market, we had some flexibility to learn as we grew. We listened to the feedback from mentors, improved our software and service, and, without any investors, witnessed Grasshopper turn into a business with $30 million a year in revenue, and just over forty employees.

My point in telling you all of this is that, in business, I've always taken risks. And if an idea fails, I'm usually never disappointed. That's because there's always an upside to doing things wrong: you can learn from your mistakes. But unlike in business, my health and wellness journey left me feeling perpetually stuck. Between one failed attempt at losing weight and the next, I wasn't learning much of anything.

After college, I became more religious about following popular dietary guidelines: consuming low-fat foods, fiber and carbs, lean meats, whole grains, lots of vegetables (which I've always enjoyed), and lots of fruit. I was also still avoiding red meat. As for beverages, I've never drunk soda, energy drinks, or any other drinks with sugar. I even stopped drinking alcohol. I was counting calories and working out a ridiculous amount. And I was rigid about all of it—I was the asshole at parties who would shame people for eating red meat, telling them it was going to cause cancer. I made sure that all of our foods and snacks in the house were low fat. Yet as zealous as I was about my own diet, the irony was that it wasn't working. Despite my efforts, I was slowly gaining weight and was always lacking in energy.

I internalized my frustration and assumed that my inability to get healthy was my fault. I told myself that I just needed to work harder. At the time, I believed that by my own efforts and discipline, I'd eventually be able to crack the code. But I never did. This went on for years.

What changed it all?

My company, Grasshopper, started to get some traction and early success. With more financial freedom, I joined a gym and hired a personal trainer to work out with me twice a week. This was beneficial, as it was the first time that I began to see a noticeable difference between how I looked and how I felt. Even though I was gaining weight due to the muscle I was building, I felt better about myself. But, this also meant I was hungrier because I was burning more calories at the gym.

At this time, the general consensus around snacking had changed. So-called experts said it was healthy to snack throughout the course of a day, as long as the snacks were low fat and low calorie. I felt fortunate that it was finally acceptable to eat small snacks at regular intervals during the day.

At work, we provided an endless supply of "healthy" snacks for Grasshopper employees. Looking back, it wasn't uncommon for me to go through four bags or more of low-fat, low-calorie popcorn per day. Snacking helped me to compensate for feeling constantly hungry, but my weight issues remained. Looking back, it's obvious that this was because the snacks that I was eating throughout the day were loaded with sugar. Still, I thought little about this because experts said to avoid fats and calories, and to exercise every day. But I was doing these things and getting nowhere.

NEVER ENOUGH

As I approached my thirtieth birthday, I'd been caught in the hamster wheel of exercise for almost a decade and still didn't see consistent results. For all the attention I paid to diet and exercise, I felt like I had nothing to show for my efforts.

But then I found something new to pour my energy and attention into: endurance sports.

At the suggestion of one of my best friends, I began training with him for the Boston Marathon. Endurance sports required a whole new level of commitment, but I was happy to devote myself to it since it felt like it could be the missing link I'd been searching for over the last decade.

For the first time in my life, I was running outside. In a matter of weeks, I went from having zero running experience whatsoever to running fifteen to twenty miles each week. Throughout that brutal winter in Massachusetts, I religiously followed my training schedule, and, five months later, completed the Boston Marathon.

Naturally, the intensity of this kind of training and calorie burning meant I was hungrier than ever, and required more food, particularly carbohydrates.

I liked this a *lot*.

Whenever people asked why I was training, I'd tell them that it was because I liked to eat. And because of the ridiculous amount of calories I was burning every day, I felt like endurance sports allowed me to eat constantly, as long as the foods I was consuming were low fat and low calorie. So, naturally, I wanted to do as many endurance activities as my body could endure.

Having completed a marathon, I decided to try training for a triathlon. And not because I was particularly excited to put my body through more, but because a new sport meant I could keep eating whatever I wanted. More training meant burning more calories. Once again, seemingly overnight, I went from having never been on a bike on the road to suddenly biking thirty to forty miles—every single weekend. I went from having never swum for exercise in my life to swimming before work every morning, and running or biking every evening. Without changing my diet, I began to lose weight because my total activity had drastically increased—even after training for a marathon!

But as I discovered very quickly, even though I could afford to eat more than ever, eating even slightly more calories than what I burned had an effect on my weight. Eating one extra meal one day would sometimes be the difference between gaining and losing weight. This was stressful, and, as you might guess, left me always feeling hungry. I was never satisfied, even though I was eating more than ever to replenish the calories I'd burned. Nonetheless, I completed several sprint and Olympic triathlons during this time, and moved on to the next thing: training for a half-Ironman competition.

Over time, though, I began to encounter something that many who participate in endurance sports have to deal with: aches and pains in knees and joints, and general muscle and body cramps. For many, this pain can sideline you from training, racing, and competing. But I wanted to do things from an activity perspective that would allow me to eat anything I wanted. Secretly, I feared what my life—and body—would look like if I had to decrease participation in endurance sports.

So I let my obsession take me as far as my aching body would let it.

I tried to optimize my biking, swimming, and running to minimize pain. I got fitted for a bike. I hired a swimming coach. I got fitted for shoes. I hired a running coach. I got MRIs on my knees. I consulted doctors. Some of this helped, but nothing alleviated the pain I was experiencing from putting my body through endless training. Despite the pain, I pressed forward to complete a half Ironman in Austin, Texas.

When the day of the competition rolled around, I should've been proud of the work I'd done. Instead, I remember the shame that I felt while changing beforehand. Here I was about to participate in a seven-hour competition, one that I'd spent more than a half a year training for rigorously, but instead of feeling a sense of accomplishment, I remember looking down at my body and noticing the fat on my belly hanging over my spandex. It didn't matter how much conditioning I'd completed, how disciplined I'd been with training, or how much I'd invested in trainers and doctors. I still felt fat, hungry, and self-conscious.

All around me were men who looked exactly like what you'd expect Ironman competitors to look like—toned, muscular, with six-pack abs. And then there was me. I quickly shook the shame from my mind and concluded that I wasn't working hard enough—that there was more that I could be doing.

Curious about the role sugar plays in your health? Check out the chapter resource at www.unstoppablebook.com/chapter2.

CHAPTER 3

THE TURNING POINT

Though I completed the half Ironman, when I tried training for another event, the aches and pains returned with a vengeance. My knees were especially bad, though every doctor I'd consulted concluded that my knees were perfectly fine. They'd suggest that I get new shoes, but I'd already done that multiple times. At that point, I was running out of options. It was then that I knew the writing was on the wall: after half a decade of participating in intense endurance sports, my body couldn't handle what I was putting it through. I took this personally. I concluded that my body simply wasn't made to endure that kind of physical activity. Today, I realize that most people's bodies—and hearts, by the way—aren't made for that kind of physical strain.

Unsurprisingly, I started to gain weight quickly without

engaging in intense physical activity. Though I'd gotten down to 180 pounds while training for the half Ironman (I weighed well over 210 pounds in college), within a year I'd steadily gone back up to 200 pounds. I knew I was burning fewer calories without endurance sports, but I was baffled because calorie balancing should theoretically work no matter a person's level of physical activity. I was still working out each day at the gym and was eating less to compensate for the hole that endurance sports left. As frustrating and scary as this was at the time—no longer having an outlet to burn the massive number of calories I needed to each week—it forced me into a new space of obsessive focus: diet and nutrition.

A DEAD END LEADS TO A MAJOR DISCOVERY

While participating in endurance sports, I'd experimented with meal-prepping, and it had taught me two things: one, portions matter, and two, the quality of food matters. These two learnings prompted me to learn more about nutrition. So, without an outlet for intense physical activity, I began to use what I learned as the starting point for my health and wellness journey for the next five years. At this time, I also started tracking my weight and body fat every single day with a wireless connected scale.

Determined to find a nutritional solution amidst the radical change in my exercise habits, I tried a wide array of things that were suggested by health experts in popular culture, like the South Beach Diet, Master Cleanse, and Nutrisystem, as well as several others. If it was a popular diet, I tried it. Thanks to Grasshopper's success, I even had the freedom to hire three different private chefs during those five years. But I struggled to get under 200 pounds. Once again, I was discouraged and concluded that it was my fault.

What else was I supposed to do? Without endurance sports in my life, I wondered if I'd just keep steadily gaining weight the rest of my life. It scared me.

But then it hit me: maybe I'd been looking in the wrong places for answers to my questions about health and fitness.

Maybe I'd been too focused on following mainstream guidelines for diet, nutrition, and wellness, when I should've been applying a more critical lens to the information I was taking in. As an entrepreneur, I'd always looked for opportunities to disrupt the typical way of doing things to drive the outcome I was looking for. But in my personal health journey, I'd done the opposite. And that was a huge mistake.

At that point in time, I started to question all of the information I came across through my research. Early on, one of the most striking discoveries I made was about the sugar industry's role in shaping recommendations on fat intake.[1] According to *The New York Times*, a so-called "trade group" by the name of the Sugar Research Foundation, now the Sugar Association, doled out cash to three Harvard scientists in 1967 to publish an article in the *New England Journal of Medicine* saying that saturated fat played more of a role in heart disease than sugar. This review, published in one of the most prestigious medical journals in the world, played a key role in influencing popular thinking about diet, sugar, and fat, and its findings were cited for decades.

Even more shocking?

One of those Harvard scientists paid by the sugar industry in 1967 was D. Mark Hegsted. Hegsted, I learned, went on to run nutrition at the United States Department of Agriculture. According to the *Times*, in 1977, he helped draft the forerunner to the federal government's dietary guidelines—the same guidelines that influenced the diet and eating behavior of millions of Americans—including me—for years.

The more I researched, the more I began to understand

---

1   Anahad O'Connor, "How the Sugar Industry Shifted Blame to Fat," *New York Times*, September 12, 2016, https://www.nytimes.com/2016/09/13/well/eat/how-the-sugar-industry-shifted-blame-to-fat.html.

the influential role big companies have on our perception of what's healthy, and what's not. Surprisingly, one of the biggest campaigns of misinformation has been around sugar, carbohydrates, and their impact on everything from, yes, heart disease to obesity and exercise. For example, when Coca-Cola began to notice a steep decline in consumption of soda, it funded research that said that sugary drinks weren't the problem—Americans just weren't exercising enough.[2]

Even more damning were reports that there was a broader play behind the recommendation of low-fat diets. According to some accounts, the president of the Sugar Research Foundation gave a speech decades ago stating that if Americans could be "persuaded to eat a lower-fat diet" because fat was deemed less healthy,[3] they could replace the fat with another type of food, namely, sugar. But some say it wasn't just the sugar industry that benefited during this time. According to a piece in the *Los Angeles Times*, "Sugar executives recognized that if Americans could be persuaded to adopt a low-fat diet, they would invariably eat more carbs. Think cereal instead of eggs for breakfast,

---

2   Anahad O'Connor, "Coca-Cola Funds Scientists Who Shift Blame for Obesity Away from Bad Diets," *Well* (blog), August 9, 2015, https://well.blogs.nytimes.com/2015/08/09/coca-cola-funds-scientists-who-shift-blame-for-obesity-away-from-bad-diets/.

3   Camila Domonoske, "50 Years Ago, Sugar Industry Quietly Paid Scientists to Point Blame at Fat," NPR, September 13, 2016, https://www.npr.org/sections/thetwo-way/2016/09/13/493739074/50-years-ago-sugar-industry-quietly-paid-scientists-to-point-blame-at-fat.

or cookies rather than cheese as a snack."[4] In addition, as the *Los Angeles Times* piece points out:

> All the "carbohydrate industries" profited from the demonization of fat, exactly as anticipated. Consumption of flour and cereal products increased by 41%, including a 183% increase in products from corn. Overall, as Americans cut their consumption of fat by 25% from 1965 to 2011, they increased carbohydrate intake by more than 30%.[5]

At this point in time, I was beginning to have serious concerns about the information about health that I'd been blindly following for most of my adult life. While I didn't consume sugary drinks, I'd certainly consumed tons of so-called "healthy" snacks made up mostly of refined carbohydrates, sometimes coated in corn syrup and other ingredients derived from sugar or corn products. And I'd most definitely adopted the mindset that sugar wasn't to blame; it was fat. For years, I'd thought, "I just need to exercise more to 'burn off' the additional calories I'm consuming."

At that point, it was clear: I needed to go back to the draw-

---

4   Nina Teicholz, "Don't Scapegoat Big Sugar. Lots of Food Producers Profited from the Demonization of Fat," *Los Angeles Times*, September 26, 2016, https://www.latimes.com/opinion/op-ed/la-oe-teicholz-big-sugar-saturated-fats-20160927-snap-story.html.

5   Evan Cohen, Michael Cragg, Jehan deFonseka, Adele Hite, Melanie Rosenberg, and Bin Zhou, "Statistical Review of US Macronutrient Consumption Data, 1965-2011: Americans Have Been Following Dietary Guidelines, Coincident with the Rise in Obesity," *ScienceDirect* 31, no. 5 (2015): 727-732.

ing board with diet, exercise, and nutrition if I wanted to feel better, look better, and live a healthier life.

NEW MINDSET

In the early days at Grasshopper, we were introduced to one of the leaders in a new area of digital marketing optimization. We brought him in to show us how to apply rapid A/B testing best practices to our marketing efforts, and it turned out to be an incredibly useful experience for us. Eventually, we ended up hiring him as a consultant to guide our growth marketing initiatives for a period of time.

Through our marketing consultant's leadership, we built a culture of learning that changed Grasshopper forever. We eventually tested everything within the business and optimized for learning quickly. Multiple times, he proved to us through his experiments that what we'd assumed to be true in terms of effective marketing wasn't backed up by the data. Whereas before we were brainstorming different marketing ideas and sinking money into them without giving them a second thought, our consultant pushed to require that our ideas were tested on a small scale before making a conclusion about their efficacy. This allowed us to focus on what was working versus making big bets—and wasting resources—on ideas that hadn't been tested. After implementing this methodical approach, the company began to grow in ways I hadn't seen before.

This iterative approach resonated with me deeply. Instead of relying on conventional wisdom to drive key outcomes, we relied on regular testing and actual data to make decisions. Years later, I wondered: What would it look like if I applied this A/B testing framework to my own health and wellness journey? What would it look like to objectively optimize my life, body, and mind with small tests, the way we were optimizing Grasshopper?

After all I'd learned about what was behind influential nutrition and diet recommendations from both prestigious medical journals and the USDA, I decided to inject a healthy dose of skepticism into my personal health and wellness research. Given my experiences with rigorous A/B testing at Grasshopper, I decided that the tests I'd run on myself would all be evaluated by the same framework, to avoid bias and make conclusions based on data. This provided the structure I needed to rule things out or in, and go deeper into areas that provided promising returns. At last, I was saying goodbye to what appealed to biased "conventional wisdom" and embracing an approach that would optimize *my* life, *my* body, and *my* mind.

BREAKTHROUGH

My experiences as a young entrepreneur in college—and then as a founder and leader of a company in my middle to late twenties—had forced me to be bold, confront fears, and learn from my mistakes. Yet, when it came to my health, I'd taken the opposite approach, relying instead on conventional wisdom to guide my decision-making. Once I realized this, I restarted my health journey with two goals: more experimentation and more data collection.

The first area where I totally flipped the script was exercise.

After moving to Las Vegas, I joined a gym close to my office. Upon noticing that they had a yoga studio, I decided to try a class for the hell of it. To this day, I'm still not sure why I went for it—after all, I'd tried restorative yoga a few years before and didn't enjoy it. Back then, I was also one of those guys who claimed to prefer so-called "masculine" workouts—things like weight lifting, marathons, triathlons, and the like. Truth be told, I saw yoga as a bit of a joke. But I'd also never taken a single class. So, in the spirit of experimentation, I changed that.

The first yoga class I went to was Vinyasa style, taught by a woman named Willow. And here's what happened: it absolutely kicked my ass. Within minutes, I was sweating profusely, using muscles I'd never used before, and—

best of all—I could tell that I wasn't further damaging my knees.

Encouraged by this first class, I went to another taught by a man named John. This time it was heated.

This class kicked my ass even more. Instead of being all about competition, I discovered that yoga classes were about your own personal flow—your combination of breath, movement, and mindfulness. John would guide us through each pose, and once he felt like everyone understood how it worked, he let us move through the flow at our own pace. Unlike when I was on the elliptical or in spin class, yoga put my mind at ease. Instead of thinking about what I had to check off my to-do list, or the emails waiting for me at the office, yoga forced me to be fully present. It had a way of quieting my mind that was unlike any other physical activity I'd tried before. It was like remembering a dance, and with each step, I focused more on my breath and the movement that would come next. And nothing else.

Long story short: I got hooked on yoga. And, like everything else, I went all in. I started practicing seven days a week and making morning yoga a part of my daily routine. I started planning business trips around my yoga schedule, catching an afternoon or evening flight so I wouldn't miss yoga in the morning, and so on. I even completed a 200-hour yoga teacher training. I just wanted to learn everything I possibly could about this incredible practice.

Yoga challenged me physically, but it was also a gateway to something even more important: mindfulness. I felt more at peace. And I even started to notice subtle shifts within myself throughout the day that went beyond the physical. I was less irritable. I was more present with friends and family. I had less judgment for myself and others, and was more compassionate.

Starting a yoga practice was a huge experiment. But it had a way of optimizing my health in much the same way I optimized those marketing experiments at Grasshopper back in the day. I started applying the framework to other areas of my life, asking myself simple A/B questions about how I felt after practicing yoga. Did I feel better or worse? Could I think more clearly throughout the day? Did my knees feel better or worse? Did I judge myself less when I looked in the mirror? On a scale of one to three, how did I feel compared to days when I was unable to practice? I logged it all as part of the process of data collection and analyzed the results.

The data was clear: something was changing. And even though I wasn't sure where my journey was taking me, I knew that yoga was something I needed. I continued to experiment with it so I could get more data. During yoga teacher training, I lost some weight and got down to 190 pounds, but I gained a bit back once it was over. But it didn't matter as much, somehow: yoga made me feel better than I'd ever felt in my life.

FUEL EXPERIMENTATION

When I was a kid, my parents enrolled me in what was considered at the time to be a "hippie" elementary school in New York City. Now they're just called "progressive" schools. Looking back, everything I learned at this school served as the foundation for approaching life with a critical lens, with the goals of optimizing for, and maximizing, learning. Through those years, I'd unknowingly applied this same approach at Grasshopper, and it helped us find great success. Somehow, though, I never thought to apply this approach to health. But with my yoga experiment, I realized the error of my ways. In order to make a meaningful change in my body and mind, I needed to apply the same lens and optimize for learning in all areas of my life. That also meant stopping the activities that halted learning: calorie counting, the food pyramid, and so many other aspects of nutrition that had been so formulaic and restricting. It forced me into a system without really asking *why* that system existed in the first place. This new learning-based framework opened things up for me physically, emotionally, and nutritionally, and allowed me to constantly learn from experiments.

With this in mind, I approached fuel—what I call the food I consume—with the same open-mindedness that had ultimately carried me into that yoga class. My new assumption was that no set of dietary guidelines or nutritional framework I'd followed in the past was correct. Any dieting strategy out there deserved a fair shot and, at the very least, was an opportunity for gathering interesting and helpful data about myself and my body.

Thankfully, my longtime girlfriend, Dawn, who had already endured the years of cooking low-fat meals, eliminating red meat, and many other "healthy" requests, was also on board with helping me experiment. Not only is she a kind person who loves to help people, but she could also see how frustrated I was with my inability to find a dieting formula that led to weight loss and optimal energy. She does most of our grocery shopping and cooking, so she agreed to get the things I needed from the store, and cook the foods I was testing with my diet. I'm not sure if she realized what she was getting herself into.

The first thing I started experimenting with was the level of my sugar intake. I'd always just assumed that sugar was okay in moderation. I loved dessert, especially ice cream. And I loved to snack. But I always made sure that the bowl of ice cream I ate at night, and the snacks I ate during the day, were low fat and low calorie. I began to notice, however, that although these products might've met the dietary recommendations of organizations like the American Heart Association, they were *loaded with sugar.*

My minor experiments led to a series of adjustments, or outright elimination, of certain sugar-filled foods. To my surprise, I began to lose some weight. When I finally cut out ice cream, my favorite, I learned how addicted I'd become to it. Even though I'd never paid much attention to sugar, especially since I didn't drink soda or energy drinks, I began to wonder if my level of sugar intake was, in fact, more important than my fat intake. That question would linger at the back of my mind as I continued my experiments for some time.

Just like that very first yoga class had sparked my desire to learn everything about the practice, my experiments eliminating sugar sparked my curiosity about nutrition, and I learned as much as I could. I also applied what I'd learned from yoga teacher training to nutrition, and began to see changes. Specifically, there were two yoga practices that made an impact on my diet.

The first was a practice called "mindful eating," which was essentially being present with your food, consciously chewing each bite, and savoring the taste and texture. This was interesting to me because, though I always loved to eat, eating had always been tightly connected to feelings of guilt and shame. I'd eat something and knew that I'd eventually have to burn the calories I'd just consumed.

Mindful eating did something revolutionary for me, though: it transformed food from a source of guilt to a source of joy and fulfillment. By meditating upon each bite of food and truly savoring what I put in my mouth, I'd engineered a truly magical moment. Instead of feeling hungry after meals where I did this, I felt full.

Yoga training was also a catalyst for experimentation with a vegan diet. A number of my yoga instructors were vegan because of yoga's emphasis on not causing pain to others, including animals. Though I didn't agree with the extremity of all of this, I figured I might as well try it. At the time I was meal-prepping, applying mindful eating to reinforce portion control, and following something of a "body-builder" diet that entailed a pretty limited diet of lean meat, chicken, and brown rice. But I wasn't losing any weight. I was determined to try anything and everything, so I tried the vegan diet for six months and lost some weight. I stuck to it, too. I was traveling a lot during that time, including internationally, which made it difficult to follow the diet, but I committed to it every step of the way. I also kept experimenting with the elimination of sugar—going a couple days a week without having it in any of my foods or snacks.

My experiment in veganism was inspired by my yoga

practice, but ultimately, I felt horrible on this diet. I legitimately felt hungrier than I had in my entire life. Even practicing mindful eating while on a vegan diet, I'd finish my lunch or dinner and feel like I could've eaten two to three times as much—and sometimes I *did*. On the vegan diet, hunger ruled my afternoon hours. With so little energy, I experienced a tremendous amount of brain fog and was extremely forgetful. All of this was significantly worse while following the vegan diet. I also noticed its effects at home: I was short and snapped at Dawn and our three children, which I didn't like. I was eating carbs, grains, vegetables, and, of course, eating vegan cookies and other things that were "safe," but all were loaded with sugar. From the detailed notes I kept during this experiment, and how I felt at the end of each day, I concluded that a vegan diet wasn't right for me. And I moved on to something else. That's how experimentation works.

After the vegan diet, it was time to try going vegetarian for a number of months. But I had much the same reaction to this diet as I had to being vegan: I felt hungry all the time and was lacking in energy. I thought maybe adding a bit of salmon would do the trick. While I still felt hungry incorporating only salmon, I felt better getting some protein back into my meals. I was listening to my body, documenting everything it was telling me, and allowing the data to move me forward and give birth to additional experiments.

Though I knew that the vegan and modified vegetarian diets weren't going to work for me long-term, I appreciated how radical they were because experimenting with them provided me with valuable data moving forward. I never tried the paleo diet, by the way. It just felt like a modified traditional diet. I wanted something more extreme. I was desperate for answers and open to anything.

As I researched these different diets, one diet that kept popping up on my radar was the low-carb ketogenic diet. This was, essentially, a low-carb, high-fat (LCHF) diet. And I was understandably hesitant to experiment with this diet at first because it went against everything I'd ever learned about nutrition. This diet didn't convert carbs into sugars for energy—it converted fat into energy. *Fat.* The one thing I'd been told to avoid my entire life if I wanted to decrease my risk of having a heart attack.

For over a decade, I'd made sure that everything I consumed—snacks and meals—were low fat, but the ketogenic diet was centered on lowering carb intake and *increasing* fat intake. The more I researched, however, the stronger this option seemed. I liked how radical it was. I liked that it went directly against many of the nutritional rules I'd always applied to my life. Those rules had never worked for me anyway, so this option seemed promising.

Still, I knew that to try a diet simply because it was radical would be a reckless pursuit. So, I set out to understand the risks surfaced by opponents of the ketogenic diet. Frankly, what I found were myths and lies cited by the diet's opponents, along with lots of gray areas, which I'll cover later in the book. Once I understood what a well-informed ketogenic diet looked like, I fully committed to it. I cut out all sugar and added lots of fat: ghee, oil, butter, cheese, all of it. I ate lots of vegetables. I refrained from snacking. I committed to my portions. Within a short period of time, merely a matter of weeks, I was feeling better than I'd ever felt. My brain fog started to go away. I had more energy. I was far less irritable. And my weight was, once more, on the decline. On the low-carb ketogenic diet, I'd eventually lose forty pounds, going from 215 to 175.

What was most striking to me, however, was that while on the ketogenic diet, my relentless hunger had disappeared. In fact, one day, I accidentally worked right through lunch. Sure, I'd skipped lunch at other times due to a meeting or traveling or something, but I always *knew* that I had skipped lunch because of how hungry I'd feel. But on this day, I had no idea that I'd even skipped it until much later.

On my way out of the office to go home that evening, I went to grab my lunch box from the sink, where I always set it after finishing my lunch (remember, I'm a man of routine), but it wasn't there. Confused, I opened the refrigerator and that's when it dawned on me: I hadn't even eaten lunch, nor had I thought about it until that moment. For the first time in my life, I'd skipped a meal unintentionally, without snacking, because I wasn't even hungry. After all the ups and downs of the journey I'd been on, it was truly a magical moment. I could sense that everything was about to change for me—that I was embarking on a new journey.

As I left my office and walked down the hallway, I thought to myself: maybe I've found what works best for me. Maybe I could lose weight and not have to feel hungry all the time. Maybe, for once, I could feel free.

Want more information about experimenting with your fuel intake? Check out the chapter resource at www.unstoppablebook.com/chapter3.

CHAPTER 4

OBSESSION

If you can't tell already, I have obsessive compulsive disorder (OCD). Those who know me or who have worked for me won't find this surprising. My workspace is always organized and my desk is always spotless. If my house hasn't been cleaned in a couple of weeks, I'll start to notice the dust building up in certain spots. I'm a man of routine and strict discipline. I fully commit to strategies and make sure that I check off every item on my list in pursuit of those strategies.

My OCD has been helpful for me in many ways, particularly in business. It forces me to have extreme attention to detail, which fuels my relentless pursuit of perfection. In other ways, my OCD has been difficult to manage. Because of the complexity of relationships, I've noticed that I'll often become emotionally distant when I don't feel like I can solve an issue. It also didn't benefit me in my health and wellness journey for a long time, as I became obsessed with the wrong things—particularly dieting and exercise—thinking that I could work harder and starve myself more to meet my goals. But hitting that dead end forced me to re-evaluate my approach to everything. And from there, I could begin my journey again with fresh eyes.

When I realized that I could conduct my own research, gather my own data, and learn from experiments on myself, I began to remove obstacles standing in the way of better health. Right around this time, I'd moved to Las Vegas. Eventually, in 2016, I sold Grasshopper, which freed up my time to pursue health and wellness research half-time. This prompted a paradigm shift in my approach to health. I had more time, energy, and resources to invest in my own experiments and learning. I'd founded a company, helped make it successful, and, most importantly, hopefully impacted my employees' lives positively by treating and paying them well. But now I wanted to pour my time, money, and energy into health, wellness, and exercise. In the same way that I'd used my OCD to optimize my business pursuits, I now wanted to optimize something else—myself. Part of this was motivated by my own personal goals, but I also wanted to help others who struggled the way that I had over the years.

Finding an exercise that worked for me (yoga) and a diet that worked for me (a modified ketogenic diet) was only the beginning. Through yoga, I no longer felt the same aches and pains in my knees and joints that came with endurance sports.

Yoga was so different: it was challenging, it was a good workout, it built strength, but it also benefited both my body and my mind by teaching me mindfulness. At the same time, my new ketogenic eating habits had prompted weight loss—at one point, before I started lifting weights again, I'd gotten down to 175. I finally felt like I had more energy than I'd ever had, I was thinking clearly, and I was experiencing less forgetfulness and brain fog. But this was only just the beginning.

Through my journey—which, admittedly, was born of my own obsession with optimization—I was able to achieve fitness goals I never thought possible: get down to my ideal weight and keep it off, improve my diet so I no longer felt hungry, and eliminate the recurring brain fog I experienced each afternoon. But in pursuing these health goals, I actually gained something far more valuable: I learned how to be unstoppable. I learned how to find a level of health that allowed me to live my life to the fullest. And I finally quieted my mind so I could be fully present with family and friends.

It bears repeating, though: everyone's version of "unstoppable" is different. We're all on our own path toward different outcomes. But whatever that looks like to you, know that it'll be the end result of a steady practice of experimentation and optimization. Fortunately, this book has the potential to make that practice much easier with the information and guidance you need to test and track the behavioral, physical, and nutritional experiments that will make you unstoppable. And with that, I invite you to begin the journey to the most amazing version of yourself possible.

You'll find more resources on yoga and related practices in the chapter resource available at www.unstoppablebook.com/chapter4.

PART II

FOUNDATION

CHAPTER 5

OPTIMIZATION MINDSET

What is "optimization"?

This word is thrown around a lot these days—mostly in business and startup growth circles, both of which I've been a part of for the last fifteen years. But as I've embarked on this health and wellness journey, I've realized how applicable the concept of optimization is to how we think about the pursuit of health.

In business, "optimization" means identifying the processes and practices that positively impact a metric you care about, for example, revenue. But in order to do that, you need data. Back in the day, business data meant looking at things like revenue, cost of labor, and products sold. With the arrival of software and the explosion of data, that changed. Within software-as-a-service (SaaS) businesses today, you can track everything. Tracking everything means you have the potential to *optimize* everything—you just need to be able to identify the patterns that help get you closer to your desired outcome.

Crucial to my health and wellness journey was collecting more data—more information about things like the ketogenic diet and new types of exercise like yoga—to get me closer to my ultimate goal. But for the first ten-plus years of this journey, I got barely a slice of what I needed in order to make a decision about what worked best for me. That's because I was relying on data and information produced by conventional thinking about health. When I adopted what I like to call an "optimization mindset" and started opening myself up to new experiences—and testing them meticulously—I took the first step toward evolving my body and my mind.

If you're serious about getting to your health and wellness goals, you must adopt an optimization mindset.

But what does that even mean? Good question.

I'll go into much more detail in the pages that follow, but, to put it simply, an optimization mindset requires that you approach every experience as an opportunity to gather data and learn from it with the goal of improving yourself in the process. In this context, we're optimizing for whatever's important to you—weight loss, better health, more energy—so you conduct experiments on yourself to make that happen. These experiments require that optimization mindset, as well as the application of the Human Optimization Framework, which takes inspiration from the scientific method: you start with a hypothesis, you test it, and you gather the results. Analysis reveals whether or not your hypothesis was correct. This, in a nutshell, is what I mean by an "optimization mindset."

In the next few pages, I'll show you how to operationalize this kind of mindset and use it to your advantage to make massive progress toward your health and wellness goals.

PERSONAL RESPONSIBILITY AND OWNERSHIP

Just like in business, optimizing your health and wellness starts with taking personal responsibility. In the world of startups, people often talk about "owning a number"— that is, owning a metric that you plan to influence by taking specific actions. In the context of your health and wellness journey, I believe the strategy is very similar. If you're trying to move the needle toward a specific health outcome, the choices you make will either be driving you toward that goal or away from it.

Optimization is about building the best version of yourself possible. It has nothing to do with being better than or competing with others. It's accepting the wholeness of who you are—body, heart, and mind—and using it to live your life to the fullest. This requires ownership of yourself and the inner space in which your thoughts and feelings dwell. It's an ownership that can position you to experience the greatest depths of life, and the many gifts you already possess, just for being who you are.

What makes optimization challenging, however, is that life pulls us in all kinds of different directions. With so many things competing for your attention, it's easy for personal health to take a back seat to everything else. That's why I've found it helpful to look at optimization as a series of small changes that we can own in an effort to hit larger goals. But before you can claim ownership, you have to do a self-assessment of sorts. It consists of these simple questions:

- Do you want to attain the best health and longevity that you can have in your life?
- Do you want to tap into your greatest potential at work and outside of work?
- Do you want the optimal life for optimal performance?
- Essentially, do you want to feel good, be happy, and live purposefully?

If you answered "yes" to these questions, you're ready to dig in to my framework for optimizing your health. It's "yes" that guides us to commit to ourselves, to experiment, and to make the most of the lives we've been given. Although a "yes" won't get us through the parts of our journey that'll be hard because they require us to abandon thinking that doesn't serve us, or habits that don't get us closer to our goals, your commitment to yourself and to living the best life possible will.

Author and doctor Charles F. Glassman has a great quote that summarizes how best to think about implementing my framework into your life: "Before I can become an expert on anything, I must first become an expert on me." The optimization mindset requires you to pay close attention to how your body responds to the experiments you're going to run in tandem with it. Optimal health, therefore, requires you to become sensitive to the signals your body is always sending in response to new stimuli. With this sensitivity comes the ability to identify when your body is functioning in an optimal state, or, as I like to put it, when you've become "unstoppable."

Why does this matter?

Because charting and identifying what's normal for *you* could be far more beneficial to you than using external benchmarks for health and well-being. For example, Type 2 diabetes doesn't occur overnight. Prior to being diagnosed, many people experience symptoms or identify anomalies, such as elevated glucose, that indicate a potential problem. But because consuming high-carbohydrate and sugary foods is common in our culture, we've normalized slightly elevated glucose readings. For example, if you feel unwell when your glucose is above 98, but the "cutoff" for so-called "normal" glucose is 100, then it'd be wise for you to consider taking the steps necessary to lower your glucose levels.

No matter where you are in life, you have an opportunity to bring your health to the forefront each day and optimize different areas of your life. You have an opportunity to find what works for you and make lifestyle choices that move your body and mind forward.

WHY OPTIMIZATION MATTERS

You can control your own evolution.

It starts with opening yourself up to new experiences, collecting data about them, and analyzing that data to understand whether or not those experiences got you closer to your goals.

Now I'm going to tell you something that would've sent my twenty-year-old self running in the opposite direction: *this isn't a quick fix or an overnight solution.*

Taking an optimization mindset with your health doesn't mean taking a prescription or losing weight overnight. Instead, it's a series of methodical approaches to the key components of health that you set in motion in order to achieve your goals.

But how does having an approach make a difference?

Three simple reasons:

1. **You'll be more likely to succeed.** Throughout my health and wellness journey, I tried dozens of diets and workouts that promised success, but were essentially designed for someone else. For example, when I replaced meals with SlimFast shakes, I'd found a short-term solution for losing weight, but I was starving all the time. Sure, I'd lose ten pounds quickly, but when I gained it all back not long after, the feelings of failure and shame returned, and were amplified. I'd beat myself up over not being able to stay on track, but in reality, I wasn't following a path that worked for me.

2. **You'll find a routine that is designed *only* for you.** Back in the day, I took popular health recommendations as the ultimate truth. Even though my body was telling me that something wasn't right, I refused to listen to it, ceding authority to so-called "health experts" in popular media. Looking back, one thing was clear: I was looking for answers. But that wasn't

the problem. It was that I was looking outside of myself and outside of my body to find them. By taking an optimization mindset, you'll stop looking outward and start looking inward to improve your health. You'll replace your lust for solutions with curiosity and experimentation. If something doesn't work for you, if it doesn't help *your* body to feel and perform better, if it doesn't clear up *your* mind, then try something else. Accept responsibility for the experiments you employ within the framework and evaluate the outcomes so that you can try something else. That's when you'll see progress.

3. **You'll maximize the potential of each day of your life.** When I was working out two to three hours a day and worried about burning calories all the time, I wasn't living. I was surviving. And I was entirely miserable. While this framework will improve your quality of life in the future, it's also about making the most of each and every day. It's not just about living longer. It's about living more *fully*.

Whether you feel overweight, tired, or out of control, moving toward feeling good and enjoying your life requires your full acknowledgment of where you're at. As you experiment, everything that you learn is valuable data, and you can use it to become unstoppable. Although it's not a rapid transformation, the small challenges the framework provides will put you on track for developing healthy habits and long-term results. So, if you're looking for a quick fix, keep looking.

But if you're looking for the ability to tap into your full potential, you've come to the right place. I'll show you how to treat your body and mind so that health doesn't feel like a chore, but rather, an investment that pays dividends.

Want to learn more about building an optimization mindset? Head to the chapter resource at www.unstoppablebook.com/chapter5.

CHAPTER 6

THE FOUR STEPS TO TRANSFORM YOUR LIFE: THE FRAMEWORK

Throughout my twenties, I was overwhelmed by feelings of insecurity about my body. I struggled with my weight and tried every fad diet and quick fix under the sun. But nothing worked.

Sure, I might've dropped some weight here and there, but it always came back. And, as I've mentioned, I was *always* hungry.

Over the years, and after all these failed attempts, I began to think there was something seriously wrong with me. After all, who in their right mind would put themselves through crazy endurance training for almost five years—just so they could eat pizza and not feel guilty about it the next day?

What I've discovered since then, however, is that I'm not alone. People are overwhelmed just like I was back in my twenties. And it's due to the fact that, in the last couple of decades, people have been barraged by competing perspectives on health and wellness.[6] From social media to celebrity endorsements and beyond, information overload has made it incredibly difficult to distinguish signal versus noise when trying to make the right decisions about your health.

But here's the thing: the noise is never going to stop.

That's because there will always be fad diets and gimmicky get-thin-quick schemes. There will always be information that sounds reputable on the internet, but isn't grounded in science. And that's precisely why you need to adopt an optimization mindset. Rather than telling you to follow a specific diet or eat only one type of food (remember my SlimFast meal replacement experiment?), an optimization mindset gives you the tools

---

6   Michelle Meyer, "The Ethics of Punking the Diet-Research Media
     Complex (and Millions of Readers)," *Bill of Health* (blog), May
     29, 2015, http://blog.petrieflom.law.harvard.edu/2015/05/29/
     the-ethics-of-punking-the-diet-research-media-complex-and-millions-of-readers/.

and the framework to make better decisions each and every day.

So, how do you start this process? Let's dig in.

START HERE

The Pareto principle is my north star—in business and in health—whenever I want to optimize something. The Pareto principle is the idea that 80 percent of your results are generated from 20 percent of your efforts.

The Pareto principle will help you to identify a starting place for your experimentation. It's an informational filter that highlights where you can invest the *minimum*— whether that's time, effort, or money—and produce the *maximum* in return. That's because your first experiments with health should be focused on producing the highest return in your health through the smallest effort.

Let's illustrate this with a quick example. Say that you're not sleeping well and have never conducted any experiments about your sleeping habits. Since sleep is such a vital part of your health, it'd be wise to run your own sleep experiment to find a way to help you sleep better. To improve your sleep, you could certainly buy a new mattress or take a sleeping pill or go to counseling—and all of these are legitimate options—but maybe, by listening to your body and evaluating your behavior, you notice that you spend the last twenty minutes before bed each night scrolling through social media feeds. Instead of spending time and money on a mattress, pill, or counselor, a good starting place for your experiment would be to try not looking at social media before going to bed. This is an experiment that could produce a significant return with very little effort. That's how you apply the Pareto principle to optimizing your health.

The goal of this book isn't to get you to 100 percent optimization and radically change your entire lifestyle. Start by getting to 80 percent through 20 percent of your efforts, and you'll be surprised how amazing you feel. I promise that if you can get to the 80 percent, you'll be better off than most people. Best of all, a lot of progress can be made simply by bringing intention, focus, and common sense into your efforts. After all, it's a lot easier to make a series of little changes in different areas to optimize your life compared with overhauling everything at once. Sure, not looking at your phone before bed might be a little annoying at first, but it could revolutionize your sleeping habits. Avoiding sugar might feel bothersome for a month or two, but it will have positive changes over time.

THE HUMAN OPTIMIZATION FRAMEWORK

In part 1, I told you a bit about how we applied an A/B

testing framework at my company, Grasshopper. This was incredibly successful in optimizing our business because it allowed us to be methodical and data-driven about where we decided to invest our marketing resources, as opposed to trying everything under the sun to generate the outcomes we wanted. It created a test-and-learn culture at the company, and it influenced me to create the Human Optimization Framework I'll outline here.

If you're willing to apply this framework to your health and wellness journey, I know you'll discover within yourself a renewed sense of health, clarity, purpose, and inspiration in life. You'll finally awaken to the fullness of who you can be and how you can feel. That's my definition of what it means to feel unstoppable.

Now, there's one thing I want to make clear: the framework isn't a specific step-by-step guide toward health. The framework is your guide for *experimentation* and *learning*. The framework alone won't get you there—you'll also need mental toughness and a commitment to putting in the work.

Here's how to begin: I recommend kicking off this process by taking inventory of the challenges, problems, or the areas in need of improvement in your life. Develop a hypothesis for how you could potentially solve each problem or improve the situation. This will form the basis of the first tests you'll run. I call this the "Identify" phase.

The second phase is called "Measure." Here, you'll be gathering the data from the tests you prioritized in the previous phase, Identify. Evaluate the data to figure out what key learnings you generated from the tests you ran.

In the next phase, called "Improve," you need to decide whether or not your findings have a negative or positive effect on your health over time. If not positive or negative, you should run another test or experiment to get a definitive answer.

The final phase is "Evolve." This is the time when you implement your positive findings into your lifestyle and routine.

HUMAN OPTIMIZATION FRAMEWORK

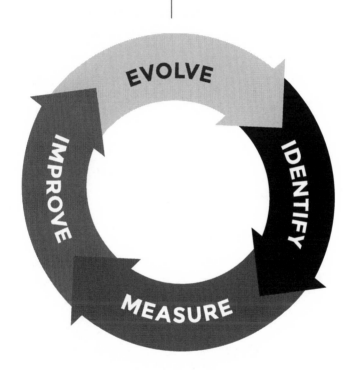

With all the information out there demanding your attention, the framework will help you narrow your focus on a single observation and hypothesis. It'll also help you organize and interpret some of the competing signals your body sends. And, because each person's body and mind are different, results will be different for everyone.

This journey isn't one-size-fits-all, so you can't compare the results you get to someone else's. Everyone is on their own path. Later on in this book, I'll share more about the thousands of hours I've personally invested in experimenting with this framework. I'll also share the science, books, research, and lectures that I found helpful and credible so you can leverage it for your own journey. But before we get into that, we need to understand the fundamental aspects of this framework of optimization through these four phases.

IDENTIFY

Taking inventory of the signals your body has been sending recently—or even your whole life—is a key part of using the Human Optimization Framework. While some of them may be tangible health problems, others may be physiological mysteries you want to solve. For example, you might have specific questions you want to answer, like, Which diet is the best for me? Or, in my case, Why am I so hungry all the time? This is *your* list, so be honest about things like bathroom struggles, sleeping problems, grogginess in the morning, or whatever ails you. Take stock of what's standing in the way of optimal health. If you don't have specific questions or urgent health issues, great! But I still recommend that you evaluate your overall well-being and performance in work, your personal life, and beyond.

Here are some questions to get you started:

- What is it that your body is trying to tell you right now? (Get specific.)
- What are the health problems that are preventing you from living optimally?
- What is it in your life that constantly prevents you from being present or productive?
- Where is it that pain surfaces in your body?
- Having answered all of these questions, what are the top three to five problems or mysteries that you would like to solve or explore?

There are so many clues that your body gives you. But, unfortunately, they're often ignored. This is your chance to be honest with yourself and take the right actions to help you avoid overmedicating, ignoring, or minimizing something that could help you live more fully.

If you're serious about discovering a solution, you'll need to record your daily workout routine, diet, actions, and what your body is saying to you. The idea here is to translate the signals your body is sending and use them as clues in your health and wellness journey.

In that vein, rather than trying to mask a problem by medicating it, I urge you to look deeper for the root cause of your discomfort. Naturally, I'm not advising anyone to stop taking medication prescribed for a serious health condition, but if you're experiencing frequent headaches, for example, it can be helpful to explore the reasons why before medicating with ibuprofen or acetaminophen. Are you dehydrated? Are you active enough? Is your mattress or office seating to blame for persistent headaches? In the long term, applying a critical lens to the medications you take will likely reduce your dependency on them, and potentially allow you to avoid many of the complications and interactions that tend to go along with taking a host of medications.

The Identify phase begins with listening and brainstorming. A lot of times, simply listening to your body can help you to hear things it's been telling you—maybe shouting at you—for a long time. But at other times, perhaps the message hasn't been loud enough, and that's where brainstorming is a crucial prompt. During brainstorming, consider any information you gather pertaining to evolution, science, and personal biomarker blood testing (essentially anything within the molecular makeup of your body that helps you to assess your health). This will allow you to narrow down areas of focus based on these types of analyses or patterns and identify the areas that could be better.

So, how does this work?

- *Evolution.* Brainstorming through the lens of evolution means considering what our ancestors did that worked for them, and contemplating what it is that we do differently. I'm not promoting a radical Paleolithic life where we walk around in bare feet and touch the ground (though this might work for some people). Just use common sense to take cues from how humans lived in the past. Maybe that means putting down or spending less time in front of a screen and more time outside. Our ancestors never sat behind a desk in a cubicle for fifty hours a week. Instead, they were on their feet, moving. This might prompt you to try standing in your cubicle or at your desk instead of sitting all day. You can gain plenty of clues about sleep, fuel, and pretty much anything else that you do in life by considering human evolution. I'll explore this concept in depth later in the book.

- *Science.* Brainstorming also means considering the research and findings in modern science. Now, I don't take all scientific studies as gospel, because each of our bodies and minds are vastly different. But scientists are smart and they're able to gather vast amounts of data that has both the depth and breadth needed to identify patterns that are worth further study. Use that to inform your own personal research into more granular, niche areas of topics that are interesting to you. For example, if you find credible research suggesting that low-carb eating is beneficial, then maybe low-carb eating is worth experimenting with. It all comes down to how it affects your own body and mind. Later on in the book, I'll go into detail about how to identify credible sources of data for your health and wellness journey.

- *Experiments.* Most importantly, brainstorming involves tracking your responses to your experiments. For example, you might be thinking about how to optimize your sleep patterns. Before investing in a new mattress, think about a smaller optimization that might benefit you faster, like a new pillow to eliminate strain on your neck or lower back. While these things may seem obvious, before I started thinking about the experiments I could potentially run, I didn't realize the sheer quantity of things I could potentially play around with until I opened myself up to them.

Now that you've spent time brainstorming, making lists, and reflecting on the numerous things you might be able to optimize, it's time to prioritize them. Since you can't test everything all at once, pick whatever experiment will require the least amount of effort and the maximum amount of change (remember the 80/20 rule I mentioned earlier). Maybe buying a new mattress for your sleeping problems isn't a realistic idea at this point because of your finances—bump that to the bottom of your list. Maybe you, like most people, can't realistically get stem cells harvested and injected into your body—bump that to the bottom of your list. If it's not attainable, it goes to a lower spot on your list, and if it can't be measured, it probably goes to the very bottom.

Ideally, you should end up with a good selection of experiments that could potentially optimize all parts of your body and mind, as well as enhance your overall well-being. This initial group should be manageable in size—so aim for around three experiments to run in a given period of time. Once you've narrowed them down, develop a hypothesis, which is just a prediction that can easily be tested. Here are some super simple examples to get you started:

"I think decreasing my carbohydrate intake by half will cause me to lose weight."

"I believe I'll avoid afternoon brain fog by doing yoga in the morning."

"I'll sleep more soundly with a more supportive pillow."

"I think I'll be more productive at work with eight hours of sleep."

This is very different from overwhelming yourself with a thousand hypotheses and trying to go all in on them. It's simple, direct, and doable. This is called an "N of 1" trial, where a single patient and single study makes up the entirety of the trial. I know that you desperately want to find an answer to the problems you've highlighted—I've been there—but you'll protect yourself from becoming overwhelmed if you stick to conducting N of 1 trials.

For much of my journey, I let my obsessions take over and was too radical in my approach to the things I tried. I overinvested in experiments and got myself in over my head with my commitment to endurance sports training. Ultimately, I ended up exhausting my body and causing it a lot of pain. But since I've started testing simple hypotheses like those suggested above, as well as collecting the data and analyzing it, the small results have added up to big changes in my life.

As time goes on, you'll find that one experiment usually creates ideas for many more, which then need to be reprioritized. I recommend giving yourself intervals during which you test specific ideas. Be intentional about collecting the data and analyzing your findings before moving on to something else.

MEASURE

Your ability to gather data and information about your experiment will become the catalyst for moving toward a solution in one area of your life and conducting additional related experiments. As you test your hypotheses, consider ways to measure your data and make conclusions based on them. Maybe you're trying to solve your sleeping trouble so you develop a hypothesis that says, "I will sleep better if I avoid looking at digital screens an hour before bedtime." Some measurement-based questions you could ask yourself in committing to this experiment might be:

- How many hours of sleep did I get last night?
- How did you feel when you woke up in the morning?
- On a scale of one to three, what was my quality of sleep?
- Did I wake up refreshed or groggy?

Without measuring, there's no way to get value from the framework. You simply get stuck in the prioritization and experimentation stages. Measuring moves the needle because you can develop new hypotheses based on the data you gather from the previous experiments. Measuring also brings another level of intention into the framework. Listening acutely to your body throughout this process positions you to track, test, and analyze your findings. Your data will most likely come in two different forms: qualitative data and quantitative data. Let's explore the definitions of both:

- *Qualitative data.* Qualitative data is descriptive. It requires you to assess how you feel or look. It's subjective, but it's extremely valuable, because it teaches you about the uniqueness of your own body. Even with qualitative data, you can generate a better understanding of what your body does in certain conditions and start to identify clear patterns.

- *Quantitative data.* This is what people call "hard data"—it applies definition to mere observations. Quantitative data includes things like blood work, weight, or number of hours that you sleep. What's important when it comes to quantitative data is considering leading and lagging indicators. Weight, for example, is a lagging indicator. There are lots of things that you can do that can make your weight go up or down (leading indicators), but your actual *weight* won't change drastically overnight.

Although there are different types of data—qualitative and quantitative—one isn't better than the other, and your analysis of either type depends on the information you're looking for. Frequently, I've returned to journals I've kept while experimenting to understand how I was feeling from a descriptive perspective when I was seeing specific types of quantitative data from an experiment. When you're measuring different variables within different experiments, some of the most interesting discoveries arise when you're testing something specific—say, if taking magnesium helps you with the aches in your joints. But then you realize that while taking supplements, your quality of sleep drastically improved. This new discovery might then prompt you to go back into the framework for more focus and experimentation around magnesium and sleep. By revisiting, this may allow you to conclude that taking magnesium drastically improves your quality of sleep *and* helps you with the aches in your joints.

At this point, you might be wondering why all of this work is necessary for losing weight, or looking a little better without clothes on. After all, that's the point, right? Wrong. With my framework, I didn't want to just *lose weight*—I wanted to learn to live my best life possible. I wanted to understand how small changes could make revolutionary differences in my mood, in my body, and in my life. I wanted to be able to explore the science behind my body's magical moments, so I could engineer more of them. To me, this is the most exciting thing about the fluidity of the framework. By intently listening to your body and documenting anything it reveals to you, you can make connections between seemingly unrelated issues. For example, when I was vegan, I lost weight, but my body was tired, and my brain fog was thicker than ever. If all I was going for was weight loss, being vegan might've looked like success to an outside observer. But by cataloging how I felt and evaluating my low energy on the diet, I could definitively rule it out as an option for me.

That's how this framework helps you find the right solution for you, and only you.

IMPROVE

Improvement requires that an experiment has been run, data has been collected, and analysis has been performed. Then you must decide, based on those findings, whether an outcome is a positive or a negative. With each new learning, you can make further optimizations and move on to the next experiment. And while experimentation can be fun, the whole point is to take your findings and make them a regular part of your routine. If, for example, taking a magnesium supplement improves sleep, or yoga in the morning improves focus at work, then it's time to incorporate those practices into your life. In time, and with commitment, those small changes can have the big impact you're looking for in your life.

Resist the urge to view new routines as binding. Remember, you started this journey so that you could learn your way to the freedom these small optimizations deliver. We don't optimize our lives for the hell of it—we optimize them so that we can spend more time doing the things we love, with the people we love, in the present moment. This creates true and lasting feelings of freedom. I mention this because there are far too many people who get addicted to the state of experimenting, where the act of trying new things becomes a preoccupation, to the exclusion of all else.

Some of the most successful people in the world report having a specific routine they follow. In this way, a routine liberates you from having to make constant decisions about what'll get you in your optimal state. That's what makes you truly unstoppable: when you've discovered the routine that lets you live as full a life as possible.

EVOLVE

Albert Einstein said that "the measure of intelligence is the ability to change." If you put these first three phases of the framework into motion, you'll position yourself for change. You'll start improving and evolving faster than biological evolution. During this phase, you should be asking yourself the following questions:

- What did I learn in my experiment?
- Do I feel better than before?
- Is feeling better still important to me?
- If so, in what area do I want to improve next?
- How can I continue to improve in the area I've been focusing on?
- How do I make my experiments a continuous loop by leveraging learnings to drive new experiments within the framework?

Remember, you're using the Pareto principle to guide many of your initial experiments, so there's no need to go super deep into one area just yet. So, for example, if you're running a test to experiment with sleep, after concluding it, don't follow it up with another experiment related to sleep. Prioritize the areas that will be the easiest to optimize rapidly. This will get you some wins early on, and it'll be key for getting familiar with this approach to optimizing your health.

For those who have been using this framework for a long time, you might want to explore certain areas more deeply over time. This is great, and will allow you to do the hard work to get from 80 percent to 90 percent optimization within that certain area. Though you never get to 100 percent, there's always room for improvement because you're always changing and evolving.

What's amazing is that, after you do this for a while and nail down your routine, you won't even remember what it felt like to feel *bad*. Your new, optimized state becomes normal, and you can continue to make progress from there.

IMPLEMENTING THE FRAMEWORK

So, once you go through the framework, does that mean you're optimized?

No. It means that your journey is just beginning!

It means that you've positioned yourself to leverage the framework in other facets of your life. It means that you've opened the door to conduct more experiments, and grow more deeply knowledgeable about what works best for you. This is a cycle that you can repeat indefinitely, but be sure to embrace the small victories and magical moments that arise when you do. They'll serve as the stepping stones to the life you want to lead, to the feeling of being unstoppable.

MANAGING THE OPINIONS AND FEEDBACK OF OTHERS

Embarking on new experiments to optimize your body and mind will be a new experience for you, and most likely, of interest to friends, family, and coworkers. While most people were very supportive of me throughout my journey, there were definitely some haters who passed judgment and responded negatively. Ultimately, for those who respond negatively, keep this in mind: it's often less about *you* and more about their own frustrations. To stay focused, minimize your exposure to those kinds of negative influences.

When it comes to talking about your journey, let others take the lead with questions, comments, and conversation. For example, if someone asks why I'm not eating bread, I'll simply give them a vague, ten-second answer, or say, "I don't feel like eating bread today." If they keep asking me questions, I'm happy to talk to them about my experiments for hours. But let *them* dictate what you share—no one likes that person who shows up at a party and proceeds to lecture everyone about diet and exercise. It comes across as self-righteous and turns people off to the transformative journey you've been on. But, by all means, be open and share your experiences with those who are supporters—those are the people whom you need the most. Be sure not to create a hierarchy around your behavior—your journey is your journey alone. What's right for you isn't right for others. By embracing this perspective, sharing doesn't have to be about passing judgment or looking down on other people. And who knows? One day these supporters might embark on a similar journey themselves.

When it comes to your household, you'll definitely need your significant other and/or children to understand what you're doing. But keep in mind—you don't need to recruit them to join you on your journey. Sure, it can be really fun when people decide for themselves to go on that journey with you, but it can't be forced. Avoid saying to your significant other, "You need to do this with me." No, they don't. That's a choice that your significant other has to make for him or herself. A mature spouse or significant other will want you to do what's best for you, even if they don't quite understand or aren't ready for that journey themselves.

Bottom line?

As long as you aren't too radical or in-your-face about your experimentation, most people will be willing to meet you where you're at, and offer support as needed. Family members might not participate in the process with you, but you can invite them to take stock of your pantry together, for example, and start a conversation about the foods that might be better for your household. If there's pushback, it's probably just fear, and your responsibility is to meet that fear with grace and understanding. Lead by example, and people will naturally follow.

Despite what you may think, this is a journey that you *can* take alone. You don't have to force others or drag them along. You can do it. The strongest advocate you can have on this journey is *you*. When you're committed to taking ownership over your own journey, each and every day, you can move forward in ways you would have never imagined.

**Find even more info about the
Human Optimization Framework at
www.unstoppablebook.com/chapter6.**

CHAPTER 7

MYTHS, MISCONCEPTIONS, AND MONEY

Antisthenes was a Greek philosopher, Cynic, and student of Socrates who once said, "The most useful piece of learning for the uses of life is to unlearn what is untrue." In other words, arm yourself with a critical lens, and liberate yourself from that which no longer serves you.

It's safe to say that when I was in my twenties, I hadn't encountered Antisthenes, and even if I had, I wouldn't have understood the weight of his words. In fact, during that time, I did the *opposite* of unlearning what was untrue when it came to health and wellness. And, instead of letting go of the practices that never served me, I doubled down on them in an attempt to punish myself for what I perceived as a shortcoming. I wasted an enormous amount of time by doing this and subjected my body to intense physical pain in the process. What I really should've done back then was abandon what I'd learned was the "right way" to be healthy, and explored what worked best for me instead.

Whether it was counting calories, avoiding fat, or replacing meals with shakes, I took popular pseudoscience as the authority on how to feed my body and lose weight. What's more, I engaged in extremely punishing endurance sports training that, along with fad diets, did little to help me keep weight off or eliminate the relentless hunger I experienced.

It wasn't until I decided to leave all of these things behind and start from scratch that I *finally* began to make progress. After that magical day at the office where I realized that I'd totally forgotten about eating lunch because I was—*for the first time ever*—not hungry, it dawned on me that perhaps everything I'd been doing up to that point might've been wrong. This sent me on another obsessive journey where I sought to understand the complexities and components within diet and nutrition—things that I'd never dared to explore whenever I was just following what popular pseudoscience had told me. At that point in time, I started obsessively researching the studies that produced this conventional wisdom and couldn't believe what I found.

It was easy to feel duped when I started learning more about all of the contradictions within the health and wellness community. But the reality is that this is just a complex area of scientific study—an area where a couple of perfect storms in our history have altered the direction of scientific discovery. You've probably experienced this complexity and confusion when trying to understand what the "right" path is to health and wellness. There always seems to be a new groundbreaking study that contradicts a previous one: fat and butter are bad, and now fat and butter are good. Carbs were good, and now carbs are bad. What's more, the science around health seems especially difficult to pin down. It's tough to know whom or what to believe. At a high level, there are four reasons why this complexity exists within research and science:

- *Human rights.* For obvious reasons, researchers can't do a lot of testing on humans. Instead, they have to resort to animal testing. And while this can be enormously insightful, it's not an apples-to-apples comparison. After all, humans and animals are different. Still, it's a shame that studies on rats and other animals are framed as conclusive for humans when that's not entirely the case.
- *Sample size.* Accuracy is entirely dependent on sta-

tistical significance, and, of course, time. Conclusive findings are difficult to produce because they require a large volume of test respondents or "sample size" to study, as well as a broad enough period of time to observe the effects of whatever's being tested.

- *Commitment to ongoing research.* Advances in our understanding of health and wellness also require acknowledgment and support from the government. After all, this type of longitudinal research can be particularly illuminating, and, in some cases, groundbreaking.

- *Economic pressures*: As I just alluded to, big business and competing economic interests make it difficult for comprehensive research to be performed. It's tough to find funding for something in a capitalist society unless it benefits the group that is funding it. And, unfortunately, those capable of funding popular research on health these days are usually big companies that want to control the outcomes, and use so-called findings to boost their brand and their bottom line.

One of the reasons I wrote this book is to help people move beyond this confusion, so they can open themselves up to taking back control of their health. In the next few chapters, I'm going to introduce you to some of my friends, who are all experts in their respective fields. With this information, you'll finally have the right information to use when applying the framework to your own experiments. Hopefully, this will allow you to avoid some of the negative experiences I had, like exhausting myself and putting my body through unnecessary strain, and then beating myself up when I didn't get the results I wanted. I can't say it enough: it's not your fault that these myths and misconceptions are so prevalent in our culture. Give yourself some grace. But now's the time to get it right. With this framework, you'll position yourself to accomplish your goals more quickly, and more methodically. I've no doubt that with a few small changes, you'll have the potential to have a massive impact on your health and wellness.

Before we go any further, here are some things you should know:

This chapter is dense. That's because I want to give you all the information you need to build a strong working knowledge of how to approach this process, and the broader framework. I recommend that you spend ample time with each section and consider how the information resonates with you. Keep an open mind, and jot down questions you may want to consider later.

It's okay if you want to skip ahead. Throughout this book, there's huge emphasis on charting your own course. So if you want to skip ahead, I totally get it. But I urge you to skim through the information on health myths that follow *at some point*.

MYTH #1: THE CALORIE BALANCE MYTH

This is one of the most destructive health and wellness myths out there today, and also, the one that negatively impacted me the most. "Balancing calories," "counting calories," or "CICO" (calories-in-calories-out) entails carefully monitoring caloric *intake* combined with meticulous *outtake*—or "burning"—of those calories through exercise. At the end of the day, it's predicated upon the incredibly popular notion that it doesn't matter what you eat, it just matters whether or not you create a caloric deficit by burning more calories than you take in.

Seems simple, right? Of course it does. That's why people love CICO and rely on this approach today. With CICO, all you've got to do is read nutrition labels, do some simple math, and commit to physical activity every day of your life.

Only problem is, CICO has massive potential to do more harm than good, both physically and—I'd argue—psychologically.

When I employed the CICO approach to my weight loss efforts early on, I found it ultimately debilitating and ineffective. Counting calories certainly allowed me to simplify my approach to eating, but it reinforced the notion that the food itself didn't matter. I could eat foods with little nutritional value, just as long as they didn't exceed the amount of calories I allotted myself for the day, and weren't more than I could physically "burn" by working out. Sure, I was eating low-calorie snacks by the boatload, but each afternoon, my brain was foggy and I was starved. When it was time to work out, I sometimes felt weak.

Worst of all, it created a cycle of shame around eating, prioritized the wrong foods for my body, and turned exercise into a form of punishment if I went too far off track.

But advocates of CICO believe in this strategy because they think the cause of obesity is simply consuming too many calories. It lends credence to the notion that obesity is due to mere overeating and underexercising. And while I'm a huge advocate of mindful eating and staying active, some experts warn that CICO itself sets people up for failure by putting them in a vicious cycle that actually makes their body demand more fuel. A person will do their best to restrict and expend calories appropriately, but over time, increased exercise requires increased fuel intake. And that's when people cave to the endless hunger, binge eat, and feel shame over the situation they've found themselves in.

In his book *Good Calories, Bad Calories: Challenging the Conventional Wisdom on Diet, Weight Control, and Disease*, writer, journalist, and historian Gary Taubes—one of the thought leaders in this space—highlights the many holes in this argument. He writes:

> All those who have insisted (and still do) that overeating and/or sedentary behavior must be the cause of obesity have done so on the basis of this same fundamental error: they will observe correctly that positive caloric balance must be associated with weight gain, but then they will assume without justification that positive caloric balance is the cause of weight gain. This simple misconception has led to a century of misguided obesity research.

Taubes says that concluding that excess calories cause accumulation of excess body fat is a circular statement. It's as ludicrous as saying that excess money causes accumulation of excess wealth. CICO works in the sense that if I were to significantly reduce my calories, then I would almost certainly lose weight. However, as important as losing weight can be to your overall health, it's *not* the only factor to being healthy. If you splurge at lunch and eat a burger, fries, and drink two beers, you're going to have to work extremely hard at the gym later in the day just to get back to even in terms of calorie counting. And if you don't get back to even, or barely get back to even, you're going to be tempted to eat very little (if anything at all), later in the evening.

But here's the thing: Your body is going to ask for more fuel when you've burned more fuel.

Most people experience an increase in their appetite whenever they're working out hard, just as I did when I participated in endurance sports. To maintain my weight while I was pursuing endurance sports and eating to fuel them, I had to keep moving the goal post with my physical fitness. And it was exhausting. And yet, this is the cycle that most people fall into with CICO. The result is a lingering feeling of having to make up for the calories that were consumed, frequent guilt or shame, and overall misery.

As I discovered, being healthy and losing weight requires thinking not only about how much you eat, but *what* you eat, too. It also means paying attention to other metrics for evaluating the effectiveness of our efforts.

Case in point? Body fat. It's much more useful to measure your overall body fat percentage than your weight because it can provide key insights into the overall composition of your body and how your organs are affected. There are many people who appear skinny, but aren't lean—that is, they're mostly comprised of fat and not lean muscle. It's a subtle distinction that, unfortunately, can have a significant impact on your health.

Despite the popularity of CICO, there's an epidemic of

obesity in the US and, increasingly, in countries around the world. Taubes makes an excellent point:

> If sedentary behavior makes us fat and physical activity prevents it, shouldn't the "exercise explosion" and the "new fitness revolution" have launched an epidemic of leanness rather than coinciding with an epidemic of obesity?

At the same time that we've been told to eat less and exercise more, rates of obesity continue to increase. While people suffer, health clubs, gyms, fitness apps, and other related businesses have witnessed strong growth: since 2000, the fitness center and health club industry has grown by nearly $20 billion.[7]

So, what's the problem here? If fitness alone is the answer to our obesity problems, why aren't we getting any thinner?

There's no simple answer, but a lot of it has to do with the prevalence of useless paradigms like CICO.

If you consider some of the more modern science about how calories are consumed and burned in the body,[8]

---

7   "Health & Fitness Clubs—Statistics & Facts," Statista, https://www.statista.com/topics/1141/health-and-fitness-clubs/.

8   2 Keto Dudes, "Gary Taubes at Low Carb Houston, 2018," YouTube video, 1:18:05, August 30, 2018, https://www.youtube.com/watch?v=cm5Cdy4-KtU.

there are much better options out there than calorie balancing. The question on most people's minds is, "What does the body do with excess calories?" Naturally, no one wants excess calories to be stored as fat. The complex view is that there are mechanisms in the body that allow excess calories to be expelled from the body via our breath and pee in the form of what are called "ketones." But this only happens if you're burning fat for energy, a topic I will discuss later.

That's why, instead of counting calories, what I suggest is a low-carb, high-fat diet. Low-carb dieting positions your body to do what it naturally does from an evolutionary perspective. In reality, fat is actually a great fuel source, and the cleanest-burning fuel in the human body because it's broken down into ketones. In turn, ketones are the preferred energy source for the brain. If you want to experiment further beyond a mere low-carb diet, I recommend avoiding sugar and refined carbs, and limiting your total carbohydrate intake. Just know that carbs from vegetables are always good because of all the fiber that comes with them. Suddenly, instead of just losing weight, you're losing body fat and building muscle—and, yes, you can build muscle by consuming low-carb foods and moderate protein.

This information will come as a surprise for some individuals. It was for me. After all, I went through most of my life thinking that feeling hungry was normal, thinking that having food constantly on my mind was normal, and thinking that snacking constantly was normal. It's magical when you realize that eating the right foods (including fats) allows you to go days without obsessing over food and feeling hungry. That gave me enormous freedom, and it can do the same for you.

These days, I no longer count calories because I know that I'm consuming exactly what my body needs to make itself productive and not store them as fat. A low-carb diet eradicated the stress of counting calories for me, and now I can exercise out of enjoyment instead of guilt. I still run every once in a while because I enjoy being outside, not because I need to exercise for a certain amount of time to burn a certain number of calories. I do yoga six times a week because I get to sweat—which feels good—and because it brings mindfulness into my life, which quiets my mind. I go to spinning class sometimes, too, because it's fun and I enjoy it, not because I had too much for lunch and feel guilty for what I ate. If your dieting puts you into a perpetual cycle of guilt, or makes you feel always stressed out, then how healthy are you? Eating fewer carbs positions my body to automatically produce the maximum return with minimal effort.

I'll discuss optimal fuel in more detail in a later chapter, but for now, simply open your mind to this idea. For a long time, this country has tried to eat less and exercise more, yet obesity, Type 2 diabetes, and cardiovascular problems continue to increase. Isn't it possible that the conventional wisdom is wrong? That doing something different is worth a try? We're an insane nation—one that keeps doing the same thing over and over again, expecting to get different results. But nothing is changing. In fact, things seem to be getting worse. It's time to try something different.

MYTH #2: THE SUGAR MYTH

Sugar is now the most ubiquitous foodstuff worldwide, and has been added to virtually every processed food, limiting consumer choice and the ability to avoid it. Approximately 80 percent of the 600,000 consumer packaged foods in the United States have added caloric sweeteners.

—DR. ROBERT LUSTIG

I definitely have a sweet tooth. Even when I got to college and became a bit self-conscious for the first time because of my weight, I continued to consume sugar. I didn't think twice about it. I was always told that sugar is okay in moderation. So, that's what I did—I consumed sugar in moderation. I never drank soda or sugary drinks. I didn't eat candy.

But I *loved* dessert.

I especially loved eating a bowl of ice cream at night, something that became an addiction for me. Ice cream was filling, delicious, and I was even told that it was borderline healthy—or, at the very least, not harmful—because the ice cream I ate was always low fat. This habit continued throughout my twenties, a decade where I was also consuming a lot of snacks while building Grasshopper. Looking back, these snacks were *loaded* with sugar. But, once again, I didn't think twice about these snacks, and neither did anyone else I knew back then.

The harsh reality about sugar is that it's not in *any* way healthy. Particularly not the way we use it commonly today—as an additive to various sauces, cereals, snacks, and more. It's in yogurts we give to kids, and coating everything from popcorn to savory foods (explain that!). The worst part is, sugar is incredibly harmful and addictive. Some studies show that sugar could be as addictive as heroin and cocaine,[9] and at the very least, acts as a gateway to other addictive substances. And yet, we continue to consume it liberally, knowingly, and, unfortunately, unknowingly. And it's causing irreparable damage to our bodies.

I say, if sugar is just a calorie, then cigarettes are just a snack.

---

9   Nicola Davis, "Is Sugar Really as Addictive as Cocaine? Scientists Row over Effect on Body and Brain," *Guardian*, August 25, 2017, https://www.theguardian.com/society/2017/aug/25/is-sugar-really-as-addictive-as-cocaine-scientists-row-over-effect-on-body-and-brain.

Still, sugar has found its way into our food supply—and in massive quantities. As the Lustig quote points out, sugar can be found in almost 80 percent of consumer packaged goods. While some people may say sugar is fine in "moderation," I challenge those same people to find a way to moderate their sugar intake when it's in the majority of the packaged goods we buy, and a majority of the foods mainstream America eats.

So, how did this happen?

There are three reasons why sugar has found its way into almost all the food we eat:

Big business wants it that way. Several decades ago, the sugar industry paid scientists to downplay the role of sugar in heart disease[10] and lay the blame on fat and cholesterol instead. When Americans stopped consuming as much fat, the sugar industry—along with many others—began to fill that void with low-fat, sugary snacks.

But why would the sugar industry bother? Simple answer: *money.*

What's more, in 2017, scientists at the University of Cal-

---

10 C. E. Kearns, L. A. Schmidt, and S. A. Glantz, "Sugar Industry and Coronary Heart Disease Research: A Historical Analysis of Internal Industry Documents," *JAMA Internal Medicine* 176, no. 11 (2016): 1680–1685.

ifornia, San Francisco, shared their discovery of Project 259.[11] According to reports, Project 259 was the sugar industry's internal investigation into the impact of sugar and sucrose on things like metabolism and gut health. When scientists performing the research went back to the International Sugar Research Foundation (ISRF) with preliminary findings and a request to continue their research for another twelve weeks, the research was abruptly halted—the scientists were on to something, but the ISRF didn't want them to make any additional discoveries.

> Project 259's early results showed that sucrose caused gut microbes to throw off the rodents' metabolisms, increasing their levels of triglycerides. Triglycerides are fatty molecules, which when elevated, can clog arteries and predispose a person for cardiovascular disease. In a preliminary experiment, Project 259 also found a high-sugar diet boosts the activity of beta-glucuronidase, an enzyme linked to bladder cancer, when compared to a starch diet. The second half of the study, which would have taken a deeper look at starch, was never finished.

It tastes good. Sugar makes things taste good. Because it tastes good, people eat more of it. The more you eat, the more you buy. Makes sense, right? Of course. Well, that

---

11   Teresa Carey, "Sugar Industry Withheld Possible Evidence of Cancer Link 50 Years Ago, Researchers Say," *PBS News Hour*, November 22, 2017, https://www.pbs.org/newshour/science/sugar-industry-withheld-possible-evidence-of-cancer-link-50-years-ago-researchers-say.

logic is what has prompted the addition of sugar to a wide variety of foods over the past few decades. People have assumed—like I once did—that as long as what they were eating was low fat, it didn't matter if it was loaded with sugar. Unfortunately, that thinking is flawed.

The complicated and—I'd argue—*dangerous* history of sugar has only recently started to garner more attention from scientists and health professionals. But, based on my research, I think sugar and carbohydrates should be avoided whenever possible. Our bodies aren't meant to consume them in the way that modern life has dictated. And now, thanks to the endless supply of processed, packaged goods, we're starting to see the deleterious effects of sugar on our health.

Evolutionarily speaking, the body was made to handle sugar from fruit in specific circumstances, small quantities, and only in limited periods of time. Today, there's refined sugar in tons of popular foods that children and families consume on a regular basis. If we're not addicted to sugar already through consuming foods like soda or candy, we're becoming unknowingly addicted due to the ingredients in our foods. It's because of all of these factors that Type 2 diabetes and obesity have been on the rise for quite some time.

To give you an idea of how the sugar crisis is killing Americans, consider these changes: the average annual sugar consumption per person has risen drastically, from 17.5 pounds in 1915 to 150 pounds in 2011.[12] This is nearly a 900 percent increase in a century. It's no wonder obesity and Type 2 diabetes are an epidemic in our country, where the average daily sugar consumption per person is 126.4 grams. What we have in America isn't a fat consumption problem, it's a sugar consumption problem. Later in this book, in discussing evolution, we'll look at how humans only started consuming refined sugars very recently in our human history, and how badly it challenges our bodies to adapt to this relatively recent development.

So, what can you do?

Here's a quick list:

- Stop eating packaged and processed foods.
- If your food comes in a container, eat other foods, and scrutinize the labels on the foods you purchase.
- Stick with eating whole foods that are as close as possible to their natural state. This is the easiest guideline to follow. You can make big improvements if you stick to this.
- Remove all refined sugars from your diet.

---

12   "45 Alarming Statistics on American's Sugar Consumption and the Effects of Sugar on Americans' Health," Diabetes Council, July 10, 2018, https://www.thediabetescouncil. com/45-alarming-statistics-on-americans-sugar-consumption-and-the-effects-of-sugar-on-americans-health/.

- Stick to eating fruit whenever it's in season. It might take you an extra twenty minutes a week when you grocery shop, but that's a small price to pay for avoiding obesity and Type 2 diabetes, among other sugar-related ailments.

The dangers of sugar and carbohydrates have been well documented and date back at least 150 years. Interestingly enough, way back in 1863, an undertaker to the royal family in England, William Banting, published a short book on his struggle with "corpulence"[13] in which he told readers that he was able to win the battle against fat by avoiding starches like potatoes. In 1957, John Yudkin advised against consuming carbohydrates in the journal *The Lancet*.[14] In the modern era, Robert Lustig, Gary Taubes, and countless others have published scientific research cataloging the harmful effects of sugar on the human body. But unfortunately, anything negative about sugar has been pushed out of popular media, or suppressed by powerful people. They'd like you to believe that sugar is okay—that sugar, in the right quantity, is perfectly safe. But, in *The Case Against Sugar*, Taubes states:

Trying to consume sugar in moderation, however it's

---

13   William Banting, *Letter on Corpulence*, 3rd ed. (London: Harrison, 1864), https://archive.org/details/letteroncorpulenoobant/page/n4.

14   John Yudkin, "Diet and Coronary Thrombosis: Hypothesis and Fact," *Lancet* 270, no. 6987 (1957): 155-162.

defined, in such a world is likely to be no more successful for some of us than trying to smoke cigarettes in moderation—just a few cigarettes a day, rather than a pack. Whether or not we can avoid any meaningful chronic effects by doing so, we may not be capable of managing our habits, or managing our habits might become the dominant theme in our lives (just as rationing sweets for our children can seem to be a dominant theme in parenting). Some of us certainly find it easier to consume no sugar than to consume a little—no dessert at all, rather than a spoonful or two before pushing the plate to the side. If sugar consumption may be a slippery slope, then advocating moderation is not a meaningful concept.

But, if sugar in moderation works, then why are we seeing large increases in per capita consumption, along with rising rates of obesity? If sugar isn't bad, why is there more dental work needed in societies where refined sugar is widely accessible compared to other societies where it's not? The evidence is crystal clear. But, like anything, when the truth is hijacked by business, the evidence gets wiped out.

MYTHS #3 AND #4: "FAT IS BAD" AND "RED MEAT CAUSES CANCER"

Two of the driving forces on my nutritional journey were the notions that fat was bad and that red meat causes cancer. Based on what I knew about health from popular culture, I unwaveringly followed these two rules. I was even evangelistic about them. I made sure that we followed these rules in our household. I sometimes made snide remarks at dinner parties to people who were eating fat or red meat. I thought that following these "rules" made me healthy. I liked *thinking* I was healthy, and convincing others I was, too. Especially since, deep down, I didn't like how I looked or felt.

In all reality, however, following these rules made me more *unhealthy*. Avoiding fat paved the way for all kinds of low-fat, sugar-filled junk to find its way into my life to fill the void. When popular pseudoscience content declared that fat was bad, the snack and processed food industries must've rejoiced. After all, they were capitalizing off of these myths, at the expense of our health.

Sometimes, to debunk information you first have to understand its origin. This is especially useful in the case of a large portion of conventional wisdom on nutrition, health and wellness, and particularly around the topic of sugar. When you start to dig deeper into something you thought was based on scientific evidence, you soon discover a much murkier and contradictory past.

To help us understand these myths and their origins, I'd like to introduce you to Robb Wolf. Robb has twice been named to *The New York Times* best seller list. A biochemist by trade, he's researched the areas of cancer and autoimmunity for years. He has always been interested in human health, but experienced a significant health crisis in his mid-twenties when he discovered that he had ulcerative colitis and was facing a bowel resection. He was following a high-carb, low-fat, vegan diet at the time and admits to being in terrible shape. As a former powerlifting champion in California, he used to weigh about 170 pounds. But on his vegan diet and with ulcerative colitis, he had dropped to around 130 pounds. He also had high cholesterol and was severely depressed.

Out of desperation, Robb began reading a book that espoused some of the same information as the popular Atkins diet. He soon became intrigued by paleo and ancestral diets, and began following both. It wasn't long before he saw immediate changes in his overall health. His digestion improved in a matter of days. His sleep improved within a couple of months. And he gained back some of the weight he'd lost suffering from colitis. As he started incorporating more animal products into his diet and eating foods with lower carbs, he began to optimize his life, body, and mind.

That was twenty years ago. Since then, he co-founded the first CrossFit-affiliate gymnasium in the world, taught nutrition education classes, and has written books like

The New York Times best sellers *The Paleo Solution* and *Wired to Eat*. Robb has graciously agreed to share his incredible insight about his learnings in the pages that follow. His work has inspired me tremendously, and he truly loves helping people optimize their lives through diet and nutrition. I think you'll enjoy what he has to say, and if you want to learn more or dig deeper, I highly recommend his books.

* * *

A BRIEF HISTORY OF NUTRITION IN THE WEST
CONTRIBUTION FROM ROBB WOLF

To distill the myths that fat is bad and that red meat causes cancer, it's vital that I give you a brief history about nutrition in the West, since this will help you to understand where some of the conventional wisdom surrounding these topics originated. What you'll see is that many of the nutrition problems we face today are directly related to what David was talking about earlier: the meteoric rise of sugar intake among Americans coinciding with the meddling of special interests and big business into our food supply. These major shifts, which I'll cover in a moment, had significant influence on the way we think about food, and how we consume it.

The prophets of the early 1800s. Thanks to the work of

people like William Banting, a popular English undertaker who found a dietary solution for his own obesity, the general consensus during this time for someone who was overweight was to reduce his or her sugar intake. It was also recommended to decrease the intake of starches—potatoes, and bread—and focus more on meat, butter, cream, and vegetables. People employed both personal experimentation, like Banting, and experimentation in clinical settings and found that the low-carb, no-sugar approach did indeed work. All of this was conventional wisdom and noncontroversial. It wasn't until the 1950s that people started to shift away from these recommendations, which were actually on the right track.

The early 1900s and the rise of industrialization. For a long time, there weren't any dietary recommendations in Europe or the United States. Dietary recommendations, however, finally started to emerge in the early 1900s when people started understanding that a number of diseases, like goiter—the abnormal enlargement of the thyroid gland—were due to deficiency issues, like low iodine. There were a number of other conditions that were caused by various B vitamin deficiencies. And so, we started learning about vitamins and potential nutrients. We started fortifying some foods. In many ways, things improved, and problems were addressed. But it was also during this time that a number of toxic things happened simultaneously, including politics getting into bed with the industrialization of our foods. There were some researchers at the time who were making some progress in studying low-fat, vegetarian diets—for moral reasons, more than anything else—encouraging people to eat more seed oils and more grains. But their findings, which were pure in origin, suddenly became politicized and economically incentivized, as the government started distributing farm subsidies with a focus on producing long-shelf-life products from refined grains.

The mid-1900s and Ancel Keys. I recently wrote a piece called "Lies, Damn Lies, and Statistics" to go along with one of my books. The focus of the piece is to highlight how everything became derailed in the mid-1900s regarding dietary recommendations (my fellow contributor, Dr. Zoë Harcombe, will explore this more later). All of this starts with the well-known researcher and biochemist Ancel Keys. Keys had a charismatic personality and was a dominating force in the academic world. He produced some compelling research about how dietary fat intake was increasing cardiovascular disease but also omitted a fair amount in the details of this research. The ideological nemesis of Keys was another researcher named John Yudkin, who was producing some fascinating research saying just the opposite of his rival—that it was sugar causing cardiovascular disease, not fat. Keys, however, was a pugnacious individual who was very outspoken and intimidating, and managed to get in the ears of some folks who were on the governmental committee that was tasked with making dietary recommendations. Keys was also one of the first academic researchers that started to use personal attacks on his rivals, instead of attacks based on facts. Because of his strong personality and research, Keys shouted the loudest, and so, his voice was heard. Amidst all this hoopla, Yudkin's research went very much ignored. The rise of Keys was an interesting confluence of some dodgy science and a quasi-religious dietary approach, along with some people having been in the right place at the right time to push forward health policy that said a low-fat (meaning low-animal-fat) diet was the solution to being overweight.

The 1960s and 70s—farm subsidies and junk food. There was a real countercultural movement in the 1960s where people started to move away from traditional American foods like steaks, animal fats, and butter—these were foods that were held in low regard with the rise of Ancel Keys' findings. It was also around this time that, in order to get elected, Richard Nixon, desperate to secure the conservative vote, promised to dramatically expand the farm subsidies program, a program that had been languishing since World War II, when farmers were given aggressive incentives for the war effort. When Nixon became president, farmers started producing a ton of corn and wheat, food that was high in carbs, funded by the government. This increase in production, however, resulted in too much food. Around the country, there were storehouses of food just rotting away. It was also around this time that some researchers in Japan perfected a process for extracting high fructose corn syrup out of bulks of corn and began to use that as a very inexpensive sweetener—something that was far cheaper than sugar cane and about one and a half times sweeter than regular sugar. Cheap and tasty. So, once again, this time period was an interesting confluence of charismatic individuals in the scientific community suggesting to the public that they reduce fat and eat more grains (as long as food was "low fat," it was deemed to be okay), the production of more grains because of government subsidies, and the subsidization of a whole process that created artificial sugar that was inexpensive and could be funneled into the junk food industry.

The 1980s—Robert Atkins and Dean Ornish. Robert Atkins, known for the famous Atkins diet, first learned about low-carb dieting from a US Air Force manual that was written for pilots who were too overweight to fly and needed help slimming down. A low-carb diet meant removing things like potatoes, bread, and beer, and eating more animal fats. For Atkins, it worked, and he became a megaphone for this type of dieting. He had a decent run, too; that is, before Dean Ornish stepped onto the scene near the end of the twentieth century, who piggybacked off of the work of Nathan Pritikin, another researcher who was an advocate for low-fat, high-fiber dieting. Ornish conducted some integrative studies where he performed some cardiac imaging on people who had stopped smoking, were regularly meditating, regularly exercising, and were on a low-fat diet. It was suggested in the imaging that they had found a formula to reverse cardiovascular disease. The problem, however, was that the error in this imaging was greater than the claim of improvement in the cardiovascular-diseased state. In other words, if you took one person and performed this cardiovascular imaging ten times, you would have little variation within each individual sample. This should have been shot down immediately—and many in the scientific community did raise concern—but once again, there was a reinforcing movement and understanding that eating low-fat foods was the way to defeat heart disease. Big assumptions were made. Counterpoints were ignored. Sugar intake increased under the banner of low-fat dieting. This was also the origin of vegan and plant-based diets that had the backing of large religious organizations and even hospitals with religious roots.

Gary Taubes and the 2000s. Gary Taubes made a splash in the early 2000s when he published a piece called, "The Soft Science of Dietary Fat," where he explored the claims that had been made about cardiovascular disease and fat intake. Taubes found what so many others had: that those claims about low-fat dieting didn't measure up to the science. His hypothesis was that the main driver of obesity—and, by extension, cardiovascular disease and Type 2 diabetes—were solely related to insulin. Insulin is mainly driven by carbohydrate intake, so he became an advocate of low-carb dieting. I think that on a prescriptive level the recommendation of a low-carbohydrate diet is really on point, in that it's a way that you can get people to reduce their total caloric intake. Taubes made some claims that calories didn't matter if you kept carbohydrates within certain levels, which I don't believe is backed up by science, and flies completely in the face of our evolutionary biology. No matter, through his work and findings, Taubes has helped to bring a number of truths back into a conversation that has been hijacked by big business and politics.

Paleo and keto, the low-carb, high-fat diets. So, in the context of this history, let's briefly touch on the two primary low-carb, high-fat diets today that I believe to be effective, paleo and ketogenic ("keto"):

Paleo. Modern researchers and medical professionals who learned about the paleo approach asked a simple question: what if features of our modern world are at odds with our ancient genetics? The so-called paleo diet concept was born through the observations of dozens, if not hundreds, of anthropologists and medical experts. They realized that hunter-gatherer groups were largely free of modern degenerative diseases. These people were remarkably healthy even despite an almost complete lack of modern medical interventions. By exclusion, the paleo diet suggests one should generally minimize or avoid grains, legumes, and dairy. Why? Because these foods are "evolutionarily novel." This means they're relatively new to our species and therefore may present problems for some people. By inclusion this means the diet is comprised of lean meats, seafood, fruits, vegetables, roots, shoots, tubers, nuts, and seeds.

Ketogenic. To make a long story short, researchers in the 1920s and 1930s noticed that patients with severe epilepsy had remarkably fewer seizures when they were fasting. That's because when they fasted, it depleted liver glycogen (a stored carbohydrate), shifting the body into a state of ketosis. In this state, ketone bodies (produced from fat) are used in the place of glucose for most energy needs, but in particular by the brain. Your brain can shift nearly two-thirds of its normal glucose dependent metabolism to one fueled by ketones, which provide a much more stable energy source. Although the ketogenic diet was born of a need to help epilepsy, many people observed that low-carb diets were exceptionally effective for fat loss. Names like Banting, Atkins, and others have popped up over the years, offering both effective weight loss strategies and controversy. A low-carb, high-fat diet has generally contradicted the recommendations of many health authorities and governmental agencies.

Now that you have a snapshot of our dietary history, I'll now break down the myths that fat is bad and that red meat causes cancer. You'll see that they're directly related to where the West has gone wrong in its scientific history as it pertains to nutrition.

MYTH #3: FAT IS BAD

The problem with a lot of the conclusions about fat that have been made in our short history as humans is that the research that has been conducted showed *correlation* between fat intake and cardiovascular disease, but not *causation*. This type of research—which is called "epidemiological research"—requires large, diverse samples be collected that are meant to reflect the whole. This was incredibly useful for the study of tobacco because it revealed an insanely powerful correlation between tobacco and cancer. The impact of fat intake on cardiovascular disease, however, was much more nuanced. The conclusions that were made about causation were irresponsible, and motivated by serious financial incentives.

Here's an example of the nuance and complexity behind the epidemiological research gathered about fat intake: in our history, people tended to eat more fat—and more animal fat—as they became wealthier. But as they became wealthier, they also exercised less and also tended to drink more alcohol because they could afford it...and they also tended to smoke more because they could afford it... and they tended to eat more sugar because they could afford it. It was true that these people were more at risk for cardiovascular disease; but this was because of the array of foods and substances they were able to consume because of their wealth, not necessarily because of their fat intake. Nonetheless, this was the only thing that was focused on in the studies of researchers who wanted to demonstrate causation. This no-fat propaganda was also pushed by a quasi-religious, vegetarian, and vegan-oriented agenda on the part of people like Ancel Keys, and then supported by shifts in governmental orientation and the subsidization of the American food supply, making for a multifactorial story as to how this "conventional wisdom" of decreasing fat intake emerged.

Reducing fat and saturated fat resulted in increases in consumption of carbohydrates, sugar, and vegetable oils. It's generally true that people have increased fat consumption over time, but what's missed in this narrative—and what's new to our story as human beings—is that fat is also part of processed carbohydrate foods: things like baked goods, snack foods, and pretty much anything that is processed, filling the aisles at supermarkets. It's much more complex than people just adding butter to a steak or broccoli. These refined carbohydrates are in the "low-fat" things that we eat. The US Dietary Guidelines—driven by the farm subsidies programs, academia, dietetics, and medical associations—have historically bought into the notion that low-fat diets are the most beneficial, healthiest ways to eat. It's a multifactorial problem.

For example, do you remember SnackWell's? It was a "zero-fat food" but was made of flour, high-fructose corn syrup, regular sugar, and some cocoa. It was the furthest thing from healthy, but had the backing of a major health association because it didn't have any fat. Well, people listened to what "experts" concluded about these foods and consumed products like this because they were endorsed by the government as healthy. In other words, people listened to the recommendations, and food producers made sure lots were available based on those recommendations.

All of this has resulted in an increase in obesity, chronic disease, and a higher mortality rate among relatively young people. Some might argue that this is primarily driven by our carbohydrate intake and chronically elevated insulin levels, which lead to insulin insensitivity, but the best science that we have at this point, in my opinion, is that people are overeating. And the drivers for overeating are these complex, hyper-palatable, highly processed foods that are high in sugar and carbs. For example, in my second book, *Wired To Eat*, I talk about a principle prevalent in the processed foods industry that I call "Doritos Roulette," the idea that within every Doritos bag are chips that taste somewhat different. You might even see a sentence on the bag that reads something like, "Caution: Some chips are extremely hot." So, some chips are hot, some are mild, and some are medium. This is intentional on the part of the manufacturer, exploiting within you what has been called the "Buffet Effect" or the "Dessert Effect"—the idea that if people have more variety in food consumption, people will inevitably eat more. You have probably been to a dinner party before where you felt completely stuffed but then still, somehow, made room for dessert. Similarly, because of the variety, Doritos Roulette makes their product incredibly addictive, which leads to overeating. Never in the history of civilization have we had so much variety so readily available to us for every meal or snack.

In lockstep with the refining of carbohydrates, particularly corn, what we ended up with was cornstarch, which was then used to produce high-fructose corn syrup and corn oil. Whereas before, butter or coconut oil might've been used on something like popcorn, they were replaced with highly polyunsaturated vegetable oils (canola oil, corn oil, safflower oil) because saturated fats and animal fats were deemed unhealthy. However, since these types of vegetable oils go rancid easily, a process called hydrogenation was developed, which could turn these polyunsaturated fats into hydrogenated saturated fats and partially hydrogenated saturated fats. The types of fats that were created through this process were called "trans fats."

Biology doesn't make trans fats other than some very rare circumstances, like conjugated linoleic acid in bovine dairy and cow dairy, which is actually a highly beneficial fat, a fat that you get from both the meat and dairy products of grass-fed animals. But those are the only kinds of trans fats that human bodies had experienced; and so, all of a sudden, people shifted from eating no—or little—trans fats in their diet, to eating massive portions of trans fats. To make things worse, these polyunsaturated fats tend to be loaded with the short-chain omega-6 fats; humans haven't historically eaten huge amounts of these either. Our biology hasn't prepared us for the direction of the food industry. So, whether they're hydrogenated or not, humans are suddenly eating an increased amount of these types of fats, which we now understand are very pro-inflammatory and cause a lot of metabolic problems. Yet they were incredibly inexpensive, fantastic in baked goods, helped to stabilize shelf life, tasted really good, and had a very benign, mild flavor, which wasn't overpowering like something like coconut oil can be. They were very beneficial in the food manufacturing scene, but ended up being a disaster from a health perspective.

Once again, it was money that was running the show and calling the shots.

Science has shown all along—with more focus lately—that natural fats that are solid at room temperature and don't require processing are actually good for the body, and might even be protective to the body. But all along, America's dietary recommendations have been derailed.

In 1961, Americans saw Ancel Keys featured on the cover of *Time*, which essentially communicated that fat was bad, dangerous, and even lethal. In 1984, it was a cover of a breakfast plate with two eggs as eyes and a strip of bacon as a frown, warning readers about cholesterol and its relation to fat consumption. And then, in 2014, it was a cover with a yellow headline that read, "Eat Butter," with a sub-headline saying, "Scientists labeled fat the enemy. Why they were wrong." If you take a closer look at the studies that were used to show that fat is bad, what you'll find is that many of them show a stronger correlation between heart disease and sugar intake rather than fat. And the truth is that we still do not have the answers, but it's apparent that conventional wisdom is far from 100 percent correct, as the *Time* covers reveal.

MYTH #4: RED MEAT CAUSES CANCER

The myth that red meat causes cancer can also be

traced back to a poor epidemiological study. The study was rooted in data from questionnaires where people were asked a variety of questions about their diet, like, "What did you eat yesterday?" or "What did you eat last week?" or "What did you eat more than anything else last year?" All the data hinged upon people self-reporting, and answering all kinds of vague questions, where their answers were most likely affected by what they thought the researcher wanted them to answer. Studies based around self-reported feeding logs should not even be considered legitimate. And, once again, causation was argued, even though correlation itself would have even been an irresponsible claim.

The claims that have been made to support this myth are interesting, to say the least. One was based on research in China that argued that, as the Chinese got wealthier, they ate more red meat, and that is why there was an increase in cancer. Once again, there could be a correlation, but causation is a foolish conclusion. As I discussed earlier, as people industrialize, they get wealthier, don't exercise as much, don't go outside as much, have the financial flexibility to consume alcohol, tobacco, or drugs, and tend to eat not only more meat, but also more sugar and more refined foods. As you can see, there are so many different factors.

Another claim that has been made through a recent study

is the connection between red meat and colon cancer. However, there is a real difference between relative risk and absolute risk. To give some background here, within the United States, everybody, in theory, has a 5 percent risk of developing colorectal cancer in their lifetime. The claim within the anti-meat scene is that eating red meat or processed meats increases your likelihood of colorectal cancer by 20 to 25 percent. But in saying this, what they do, for the sake of making headlines and portraying things as scarier than they actually are, is ignore the absolute risk.

Well, guess what?

The difference between 5 percent and 6 percent is about 20 percent—this is the distortion that can happen when you alternate between absolute and relative numbers. That is to say, it's easy to make a number sound very large by quoting the percentage increase or decrease. In this case, to go from 5 percent to 6 percent would most likely entail consuming large amounts each day for the rest of your life, which virtually no one does. A lot of these studies have clear motives behind them from proponents of vegan and plant-based diets, which have become socially connected with morality and a lot of money behind these campaigns to influence popular culture.

A related claim has also been made that eating animals

is not only bad for people but is also bad for the environment. Addressing this claim can be a daunting task, as many who challenge this notion—one that, by the way, is directly related to global warming—are immediately viewed as right-wing wackos who are ignorant of science. Hopefully you can tell by now that I'm actually trying to keep the science accountable and point out the legitimate flaws in a lot of the claims that have been made. So, to dive in, there's a claim that the production of animal products is a big vector for the different types of greenhouse gases, carbon dioxide, and methane. There's some truth to that. But this is mainly in the context of the industrialized feedlot process. When they put cows on the feedlot system, what they're doing is feeding them grains—and these grains have been grown using fossil fuels.

How this works is that farmers grow corn, wheat, barley, or whatever it may be; it gets raised; it gets processed; it gets shipped around the country or around the world; and then the leftovers get put into these feedlots. But when you look at the flip side of this and consider a holistically managed practice of raising ruminants on grass, you have a very tight loop: the sun shines on the grass, the grass sequesters carbon dioxide and other nutrients, those nutrients grow, and then ruminants—animals with two stomachs and a biological process made to break down vegetation that humans can't consume—eat the grass and also grow. And then, eventually, they're either eaten by humans or predators—or the animal just dies.

When you look at the total energy input and carbon footprint of pastured meat, and holistically managed meat, in animal products, it is completely different than that which is used in conventional animal husbandry. Part of what happens when the plants are taking in sunlight and using carbon dioxide and water to make sugars and starch is that the sugar and starch goes underground and feeds bacteria and fungus. This is soil. Part of what the fungus does is mine minerals that it shares with the bacteria, which it then shares with the plants. And so, in these areas where there are grasslands, like in the steppes of Siberia, which are very similar to the North American grasslands, the roots of these plants can sometimes venture hundreds of feet into the ground. The American Plains used to have hundreds of feet of topsoil, and now it's down to about twelve to fifteen feet of topsoil because of conventional farming practices, which are row-crop based, which is the centerpiece of the vegan diet—comprised of grains and legumes. The way that grains and legumes are grown is unsustainable in row-crop fashion. So, the irony is that a vegan's recommendation would accelerate climate change and accelerate the loss of topsoils. The United Nations put out a report suggesting that the world at large has sixty years of topsoil left. And, once the topsoil is gone, our ability to feed ourselves would effectively be gone.

But, if people understood the way that this holistic management could occur, we could be producing huge amounts of food and sequestering carbon, potentially returning carbon levels to pre-industrialized atmospheric levels in this virtuous cycle of food production and soil restoration. But, it's a really complex story, and it is virtually political suicide to even suggest that you could use effective animal husbandry to address climate change. Anyway, all of this is related to the myth that red meat causes cancer and that eating animals is bad for both humans and the environment.

* * *

MYTH #5: THE FAT MYTH (CONTINUED)

For some of you, this might be your first time even considering that fat *isn't* bad. Don't worry. When I was first exposed to the idea that fat might not be bad after all, I struggled to believe it, too. It was one of my core dieting principles that had dictated how I ate for such a long time. Especially when I started experimenting with a low-carb, high-fat diet, and started seeing immediate results, it almost felt too good to be true. I obsessively researched all kinds of different arguments about fat, weighing all the data and making sure that I was approaching something that felt so radical with a level head. What I discovered, at the very least, was what Robb Wolf communicated earlier: that conventional wisdom was unequivocally wrong in its certainty about the perils of fat. There had been far too much politics, nuance, and confusion around the issue to make a conclusion.

But because there is so much confusion around the role of fat in our nutrition, I wanted to include a second voice on this topic, Dr. Zoë Harcombe, who has a PhD in public health nutrition. Zoë, also a published author, has impacted my journey much the same way Robb Wolf has. In the section that follows, Zoë takes things deeper, especially for those of you who are skeptical or worried about suddenly changing your diet and consuming more fat. Here, we venture deeper into the science and data supporting the claims made. Zoë has dedicated much of her life to attempting to answer the question, "Why is there still an obesity problem when people so desperately want to be slim?" Her life goal is to eradicate the obesity epidemic. She published her first book in 2004, titled *Why Do You Overeat? When All You Want Is to Be Slim*, and has published several books and academic articles since. It's an honor to include such a brilliant mind in this book.

In focusing on the data that was available at the time that the dietary fat guidelines emerged, and the new data that has come out since then, Zoë has deciphered the real story behind the numbers. As maddening as all of this is, her perspective is both eye-opening and helpful in figuring out how we got to this point.

* * *

THE DEMONIZATION OF DIETARY FAT: THE SHORT STORY

CONTRIBUTION FROM DR. ZOË HARCOMBE

At a time when science plays such a powerful role in the life of society, when the destiny of the whole of mankind may hinge on the results of scientific research, it is incumbent on all scientists to be fully conscious of that role and conduct themselves accordingly.

—JOSEPH ROTBLAT

Science is the great antidote to the poison of enthusiasm and superstition.

—ADAM SMITH, *THE WEALTH OF NATIONS*, 1776

Agencies involved in public health are responsible for providing the populace with the information necessary to make choices that will optimize well-being. Nutrition guidelines are one aspect of public health, as are the well-known directives to stop smoking and to avoid excessive alcohol and sedentary lifestyles. Like all medical specialties, public health is expected to provide evidence-based recommendations, not ideology. But expectations don't always reflect reality. And so begins a story that needs to be told—the story of how dietary fat became the bogey-man held responsible for the millions of people afflicted with heart disease. The plot twist? Dietary fat wasn't the problem after all.

A QUICK PRIMER ON DIETARY FAT AND DIETARY FAT GUIDELINES

To critically evaluate the conventional wisdom that "fat is bad," it's essential to have at least a basic understanding of dietary fat. First, dietary fats are vital for human life. Fats provide fat-soluble vitamins and the essential fatty acids omega-3 and omega-6. Secondly, all foods that contain fat (meat, fish, eggs, dairy, nuts, seeds, avocados, olives, grains, legumes, etc.) provide a mix of saturated, polyunsaturated, and monounsaturated fat. That is true for foods of both plant and animal origin. Except for dairy products, all food groups have more unsaturated than saturated fat and, yes, that includes meat.

Knowing that foods contain a mix of fats is just one reason to reject the notion that saturated fat is harmful and unsaturated fat is healthful—why would nature always provide them together if this were the case? The facts about fat also dispel the myth that animal products are synonymous with saturated fat and plant foods with unsaturated fat. Any food with fat, of plant or animal origin, will contain saturated and unsaturated fat. Coconut oil is vegan, but it also happens to have the highest saturated fat content of any single food.

To return to someone, Dr. Ancel Keys, it's important to understand just how hugely influential he was when it came time for the US and UK governments to establish dietary guidelines in the late 1970s and early 1980s. The work of Dr. Keys provided, in large part, the rationale for the 1980 American dietary guidelines, and the 1984 UK dietary guidelines.

The guidelines recommended that total fat was to be limited to 30 percent of caloric intake, and saturated fat was to contribute no more than 10 percent of daily calories.[15] [16] In a natural diet, protein is relatively constant at about 15 percent of daily calories. As a result, limiting fat to a maximum of 30 percent means that carbohydrates would provide at least 55 percent of the daily caloric intake. Thus emerged the low-fat, high-carbohydrate diet that has been embraced by millions since. This same diet also spurred the food industry to manufacture products like low-fat ice cream, fat-reduced salad dressings, and potato chips that were "baked, not fried."

15 Select Committee on Nutrition and Human Needs. Dietary Goals for the United States (Washington: U.S. Govt. Print. Off., February 1977).

16 National Advisory Committee on Nutritional Education (NACNE). "A Discussion Paper on Proposals for Nutritional Guidelines for Health Education in Britain," 1983.

The dietary fat guidelines (DFGs) adopted by the UK and the US influenced a great number of other countries to model their approach to nutrition around the 30/10 "rule." In other words, these guidelines, driven, as discussed here, by something other than rigorous scientific evidence, have had an impact on a worldwide scale.

Undertaking a meta-analysis of the data that was available before recommendations were introduced certainly raises red flags about the willingness of governmental bodies to give the DFGs their stamp of approval. Starting with a meta-analysis of the six RCTs available prior to the 30/10 limits being entrenched in nutrition guidelines, the findings were as follows:[17]

- Dietary fat interventions did not result in any statistically significant difference in coronary heart disease (CHD).
- These same interventions also did not result in any difference in all-cause mortality.
- Individually, none of these studies recommended the DFGs that were subsequently adopted. In fact, one study went as far as to state, "A low-fat diet has no place in the treatment of the myocardial infarction."[18]

---

17 Z. Harcombe et al., "Evidence from Randomised Controlled Trials Did Not Support the Introduction of Dietary Fat Guidelines in 1977 and 1983: a Systematic Review and Meta-analysis," *Open Heart* 2, no. 1 (2015), doi: 10.1136/openhrt-2014-000196.

18 Research Committee, "Low-fat Diet in Myocardial Infarction: A Controlled Trial," *The Lancet* 2, no. 7411 (1965): 501-4.

- None of the studies specifically looked at the impact of simultaneously limiting total fat to 30 percent and saturated fat to 10 percent. In other words, the recommended total and saturated fat percentages were determined by extrapolation and conjecture rather than being determined by RCTs.

Due to the nature of their data, the epidemiological studies available before September 1983 were not suitable for a meta-analysis. However, a systematic review of the six epidemiological studies available prior to 1983 identified the following:[19]

- Five studies found no statistical association between total or saturated fat and deaths from CHD.
- One study found a statistically significant association between saturated fat (but not total fat) and CHD. This study is referred to as the Seven Countries Study (SCS) and was authored by Dr. Keys, et al.[20] [21]
- Overall, the epidemiological studies clearly did not support the introduction of the 30/10 DFGs.

---

19 Z. Harcombe, J.S. Baker, and B. Davies, "Evidence from Prospective Cohort Studies Did Not Support the Introduction of Dietary Fat Guidelines in 1977 and 1983: a Systematic Review," *British Journal of Sports Medicine* (2016), doi: 10.1136/bjsports-2016-096409.

20 A. Keys, "Coronary Heart Disease in Seven Countries I. The Study Program and Objectives," *Circulation* 41 (1970), doi: 10.1161/01.CIR.41.4S1.I-1.

21 A. Keys, *Seven Countries: a Multivariate Analysis of Death and Coronary Heart Disease* (Harvard University Press, 1980).

The Seven Countries Study is worth examining in greater detail, as there are several reasons why the data needs to be interpreted with caution. These reasons include the following:

- As an epidemiological study, any associations cannot be considered evidence of causation.
- The study excluded women, and did not exclude men with documented heart disease. It also only examined men within a specific age range (ages forty to fifty-nine). As such, the results are not generalizable to the general population, the target of the DFGs.
- The study did not find an association between heart disease and other known risk factors, including smoking, weight, and sedentary behavior. This alone raises concerns about the accuracy of the findings.
- The dietary information used to conclude that saturated fat is associated with CHD was only collected from just over 3 percent of the participants. Further, these data were based on subject (and wife) recall, a notoriously unreliable source of information.
- And, the most concerning of all, the SCS was an inter- (rather than intra-) country study. What this means is that countries were compared to each other rather than comparing people within a single country. In other words, the Finnish men who developed CHD were compared to American men who developed CHD rather than comparing the diet intake of American

men who did or did not develop CHD. An inter-country comparison does not consider a multitude of differences between countries that could, in and of themselves, explain differences in heart health. For example, the local healthcare system, latitude (with its influence on vitamin D levels), GDP, climate, and characteristics of the country's typical diet, can all have significant associations with health, CHD included.

Of note, one of the statistically significant findings from the SCS was that the death rate for men with previous heart disease was close to 21 percent, compared to a death rate of 1 percent for men without such a history. This finding underscored a very significant risk factor for dying from heart disease: having it in the first place. This finding wasn't emphasized, with the authors instead focusing on the association between saturated fat and CHD.

THE EVIDENCE SINCE THEN

The evidence that has accrued since the introduction of the DFGs has not offered any additional support for the 30/10 recommendations. When a systematic review and meta-analysis of relevant RCTs was undertaken, these were the key findings:[22]

---

22 Z. Harcombe, J.S. Baker, J.J. DiNicolantonio, F. Grace, and B. Davies B,. "Evidence from Randomised Controlled Trials Does Not Support Current Dietary Fat Guidelines: a Systematic Review and Meta-analysis," *Open Heart* 3, no. 2 (2016), doi: 10.1136/openhrt-2016-000409.

- Dietary fat interventions did not significantly change the number of deaths from CHD or all causes.
- The evidence does not support the 30/10 DFGs.

A similar analysis of relevant epidemiological studies found the following:[23]

- Total fat is not associated with deaths due to heart disease.
- Saturated fat is not associated with deaths due to heart disease.
- The evidence does not support the 30/10 DFGs.

While it is true that there are individual epidemiological studies that have found an association between total and saturated fat and CHD, there are as many that haven't. Many of these studies suffer from their own shortcomings, and none could establish causation anyway. The gold standard remains systematic review and meta-analyses, the results of which do not support the recommendation that the populace abides by the 30/10 limits in pursuit of better cardiovascular health.

Surprisingly, research both before and after the introduction of the DFGs rarely specifically tested the 30/10

23 Z. Harcombe, J. Baker, and B. Davies, "Evidence from Prospective Cohort Studies Does Not Support Current Dietary Fat Guidelines: A Systematic Review and Meta-analysis," *British Journal of Sports Medicine* (2016), doi:10.1136/bjsports-2016-096550.

guidelines. There have been a few studies that have examined specific percentages but none that were 100 percent congruent with the 30/10 target. For example:

- The STARS study (1992) looked at a total fat intake of 27 percent and a saturated fat intake of 8 to 10 percent. This very small study (fifty-five men) was the closest to the DFG of 30/10.[24]
- The DART (1989) study tested 30 percent total fat, but this trial was confounded by an effort to make polyunsaturated and saturated fat intake equal.[25]
- Two RCTs looked at a 20 percent fat diet.[26] [27]
- Two other studies looked at 10 percent saturated fat but without the 30 percent limit on total fat.[28] [29] (It's also worth noting that one of the studies that limited

24 G. F. Watts et al., "Effects on Coronary Artery Disease of Lipid-Lowering Diet, or Diet Plus Cholestyramine, in the St Thomas' Atherosclerosis Regression Study (STARS)," *The Lancet* 339, no. 8793 (1992): 563-9.

25 M.L. Burr, et al., "Effects of Changes in Fat, Fish, and Fibre Intakes on Death and Myocardial Reinfarction: Diet and Reinfarction Trial (DART)," *The Lancet* 2, no. 8666 (1989): 757-61.

26 Research Committee, "Low-fat Diet in Myocardial Infarction: A Controlled Trial," *The Lancet* 2, no. 7411 (1965): 501-4.

27 B.V. Howard et al., "Low-fat Dietary Pattern and Risk of Cardiovascular Disease: the Women's Health Initiative Randomized Controlled Dietary Modification Trial," *JAMA* 295, no. 6 (2006): 655-66, doi: 10.1001/jama.295.6.655.

28 J.M. Woodhill, A.J. Palmer, B. Leelarthaepin, C. McGilchrist, and R.B. Blacket, "Low Fat, Low Cholesterol Diet in Secondary Prevention of Coronary Heart Disease." *Advances in Experimental Medicine and Biology* 109 (1978): 317-30.

29 I.D. Frantz, et al., "Test of Effect of Lipid Lowering by Diet on Cardiovascular Risk. The Minnesota Coronary Survey," *Arteriosclerosis, Thrombosis, and Vascular Biology* 9, no. 1 (1989): 129-35, doi: 10.1161/01.atv.9.1.129.

saturated to fat to 10 percent found that the death rate increased!)

The inescapable conclusion is that dietary recommendations related to fat intake were adopted, promoted, and defended in the absence of rigorous scientific evidence. Good intentions led to misguided actions, and citizens (and their health) have suffered accordingly. The 1977–1983 dietary fat guidelines were undoubtedly a turning point in population nutrition—just not a good one.

PUTTING IT ALL TOGETHER

The bottom line is this: the evidence available before and after the dietary fat guidelines were introduced does not support the "dietary fat leads to heart disease" hypothesis. Likewise, the evidence does not support the 30/10 recommendations that flowed from this hypothesis.

Our research group is not the only one that has conducted meta-analyses on the topic. In looking at a group of eight meta-analyses (including one from our work), the results are astonishing.[30] Thirty-five of the thirty-nine findings were not statistically significant—in other words, they did not support the introduction of the DFGs. Further, the

---

30 Z. Harcombe, "Dietary Fat Guidelines Have No Evidence Base: Where Next for Public Health Nutritional Advice?" *British Journal of Sports Medicine* (2016) doi: 10.1136/bjsports-2016-096734.

four studies that at first glance did find a link between dietary fat and CHD [31] [32] [33] [34] had either obvious shortcomings (e.g., including poor quality research, excluding higher quality studies) or examined trans fat, a nutrient not even included in the 30/10 guidelines. The bottom line is this: the high-quality, easily defensible evidence that must be available to justify population-wide dietary guidelines such as the 30/10 recommendations is simply nowhere to be found.

The one ostensibly significant finding reported in 2011 and 2015 did not reflect studies of healthy people of both genders. So again, this claim (which did not withstand testing) is not generalizable to the public at large, the intended audience for the DFGs.

In the end, the four out of thirty-nine findings that initially purported to support the DFGs are either not relevant (the trans fat study) or arose from studies that have

---

31 R. Chowdhury et al, "Association of Dietary, Circulating, and Supplement Fatty Acids With Coronary Risk: A Systematic Review and Meta-analysis," *Annals of Internal Medicine* 160, no. 6 (2014): 398-406, doi: 10.7326/M13-1788.

32 D. Mozaffarian, R. Micha, and S. Wallace, "Effects on Coronary Heart Disease of Increasing Polyunsaturated Fat in Place of Saturated Fat: a Systematic Review and Meta-analysis of Randomized Controlled Trials," *PLoS Medicine* 7 (2010).

33 L. Hooper et al., "Reduced or Modified Dietary Fat for Preventing Cardiovascular Disease," *Cochrane Database of Systematic Reviews (Online)* 7 (2011): CD002137, doi: 10.1002/14651858. CD002137.pub2.

34 L. Hooper, N. Martin, A. Abdelhamid, and G. Davey Smith, "Reduction in Saturated Fat Intake for Cardiovascular Disease," *Cochrane Database of Systematic Reviews* 6 (2015), doi: 10.1002/14651858.CD011737.

apparent shortcomings. In the latter case, the findings are simply not examples of the high-quality, easily defensible evidence that must be in place to justify population-wide dietary guidelines such as the DFG.

So, how does one explain why the dietary fat guidelines were embraced so readily and for so long despite there being so much evidence to the contrary? One possible explanation is that the guidelines were an example of governmental reactivity rather than government responsiveness to the best evidence available. The reactivity reflected the perceived costs; for example, mortality, morbidity, and financial burden of heart disease. Although, as noted before, a CHD annual death rate of 0.59 percent would not be considered a crisis by many. Maybe things weren't so desperate after all. Essentially, Keys and his supporters argued that "something had to be done," and it was.

The dietary guidelines were embraced, changes were made in the food industry and in the healthcare system, and yet heart disease continues to plague the developed world. Certainly, reductions in death rates have occurred, but these can be explained by parallel reductions in smoking and in improved access to emergency "heart attack" care. However, there is no evidence that changes resulting from the dietary guidelines have had an impact. The RCTs confirmed this—even where interventions did have an effect—that is, interventions that successfully reduced serum cholesterol, the critical endpoint—deaths related to heart disease didn't budge. Clearly, interventions based on the dietary fat → serum cholesterol → heart disease paradigm have not accomplished the stated goals. Predictably, given what the research said even before their adoption, the 30/10 guidelines haven't, and won't, solve the heart disease problem.

Not only did the DFGs fail to achieve the intended results, but they also had other deleterious effects. By demonizing foods based on their "high" fat content, the intake of meat, nuts, cheese, eggs, and the like, was discouraged. As the public attempted to curtail the amount of fat in their diet, space opened on the average dinner plate. That space was readily filled with carbohydrates—think pasta, noodles, rice, fries, instant mashed potatoes, and bread (unbuttered, of course)—indeed, the guidelines mandated this. We know now that as carbohydrates became a more significant part of the diet, high blood sugar and obesity became a more significant public health problem in the UK, the US, and well beyond.[35] [36] Sadly, it seems that by paving the way for increased carbohydrate intake, the 30/10 DFGs may have contributed to the Type

---

35 Michael Wadsworth, Diana Kuh, Marcus Richards, and R. Hardy, "Cohort Profile: The 1946 National Birth Cohort (MRC National Survey of Health and Development)," *International Journal of Epidemiology* 35 (2006): 49-54, doi: 10.1093/ije/dyi201.

36 Centers for Disease Control and Prevention, "Long Term Trends in Diabetes. In: *Translation CDoD*, ed. (Centers for Disease Control and Prevention, October 2014).

2 diabetes pandemic gripping so many countries. Further, focusing on dietary fat as the cause of heart disease has resulted in wasted time, effort, and money that could otherwise have been used to develop and implement nutrition recommendations genuinely based on rigorous scientific evidence.

LESSONS LEARNED

Good intentions notwithstanding, the dietary fat guidelines that have been perpetuated both formally and informally since 1977 were not an accurate reflection of the evidence available at the time or the evidence available since then. High-level analyses of available studies do not support the contention that dietary fat intake contributes significantly to heart disease and related outcomes.

It's time to revise the dietary fat/heart disease paradigm to reflect the evidence available. It's also time to consider the possibility that saturated fat has never been the issue, but that the company it keeps in highly processed foods may be. In other words, saturated fat from natural, whole foods (eggs, meat, dairy, avocados, and even olives) is not a concern. Processed foods that contain saturated fat (cookies, pizza, muffins, ice cream, etc.) may be worth further examination, but not because of the fat content. Instead, it may be the carbs and trans fat found in those types of foods that pose the real threat to population health. Saturated fat has simply been a victim of guilt by association.

Science has the power to inform, but it also has the power to sway in the wrong direction if it isn't objectively and critically evaluated. When the stakes are so high—when population and personal health can be guided or misguided by available science—careful attention must be paid to the quality of research. When that attention is applied, albeit long past due, the dietary fat → heart disease hypothesis remains unproven. Thus, the 2015 US guidelines took a step in the right direction, removing the recommendation to limit dietary cholesterol and removing the 30 percent total fat recommendation. The 10 percent limit for saturated fat remains, and we strongly argue that this decision should be re-examined in light of the evidence presented in this chapter.

Government guidelines and professional practice don't always change quickly in response to new (or old) evidence. Thankfully, individuals don't have to be burdened by a pace of change that can approach inertia. The available evidence provides more than enough rationale to rethink the "fat is bad for your heart" mantra that has been repeated for years. Rejecting this demonization of dietary fat is a crucial step in developing nutrition recommendations that can genuinely help the public achieve and maintain optimal health.

* * *

The Dietary Guidelines for Americans (DGA) in 1980 misled Americans in catastrophic ways. Since then, rates of Type 2 diabetes have quadrupled, and the rate of adult obesity has nearly doubled. These skyrocketed because the American people were misinformed about what a healthy diet looked like, as they were encouraged by the DGA to shift away from consuming fat- and protein-based foods toward ridiculous amounts of carbohydrate-based foods. This became even more complicated when, with the rapid increase in obesity over the last three and a half decades, Americans were fed another lie: that weight loss hinges upon exercise, when, in fact, it actually hinges upon diet. Though it's impossible to ever do enough work to make up for the damage that has been done with this health crisis, people like Robb and Zoë, along with organizations like the Nutrition Coalition, are trying to get the correct information out there and help Americans to learn from the DGA's past sins. As daunting and discouraging as it can feel to confront these lies, applying the framework and adopting an optimization mindset opens up the gates of opportunity. A few shifts in this area can change everything in your health moving forward.

MYTH #6: THE CHOLESTEROL MYTH

When I first started experimenting with a high-fat, low-carb diet, my biggest concern was cholesterol. Yes, I felt better than ever. I was losing weight. I finally wasn't hungry all the time. But was it worth it if I were only to discover an astronomical increase in my cholesterol? I knew that following a high-fat diet would inevitably increase my cholesterol, which had long been linked to cardiovascular disease, so I couldn't help but wonder: was this newfound diet going to kill me?

At the same time, conventional wisdom had been wrong in its certainty about the importance of low-fat foods, its tolerance of sugar, and its avoidance of red meat and fat, so could it be possible that it was *also* wrong about high cholesterol levels being linked to cardiovascular disease? Before I went any further in pursuing a high-fat, low-carb diet, I gathered information for myself about cholesterol, curiously exploring whatever would be useful to me on my own journey.

Though I sifted through a wide array of research and science from all over the spectrum related to cholesterol, the most impactful information came from a man named Ivor Cummins, host of *The Fat Emperor* podcast and regular speaker on the topics of diabetes and heart disease. What I found especially interesting about Ivor's work was the fact that he isn't a traditional diet or health researcher.

He's an engineer by trade, with a degree in chemical engineering and specialization in complex problem-solving methodology, an obsession with root cause analysis, a term more typically used in software engineering, but applicable to almost any other scenario. Ivor, like Robb, began his research for personal reasons, which mirrored my own journey of experimentation. Upon receiving a blood test with poor results, he began to study the causes of dyslipidemia, the name for abnormally high cholesterol or fats in the bloodstream. As he studied the causes behind his negative blood test, he realized that the research required far more than a generic medical background to determine the origin of this common disease. It, in fact, required analysis by someone with deep experience in root cause analysis, something with which Ivor was extremely familiar.

Ivor started out hoping to find answers to his elevated levels of cholesterol, but instead, he stumbled upon something far more complex: the systematic denial of sugar's powerful role in heart disease. As Ivor has pointed out in many talks and podcast episodes, insulin resistance plays a much more powerful role in the risk of cardiovascular disease than cholesterol does, and that insulin resistance is caused by the consumption of huge quantities of sugar that the human body isn't able to process. What's more, Ivor contends—as I do—that the best indicator of potential heart disease isn't your cholesterol number, it's your coronary artery calcium (CAC) results. Although few people are familiar with the CAC scan, in 2018, the American Heart Association/American College of Cardiology broadly endorsed the test for at-risk patients.[37] But it's probably useful for a much broader segment of the population, particularly those who are trying to parse signal versus noise when it comes to cardiovascular health.

You can do more to decrease your risk of cardiovascular disease by cutting out sugar and carbohydrates than worrying about your levels of cholesterol from eating fat. This isn't just a trendy conclusion—it's proven by ample scientific and medical research that has been systematically buried.

But why, you might ask, why would anyone bury this type of useful data?

The simple answer is money.

The more complex one is: people make more money by *avoiding* determining the actual root cause of heart disease and charging patients and insurance to patch the problems around it than by solving the root cause of heart

---

37 "The Heart Test You May Need—But Likely Haven't Heard Of," Johns Hopkins Medicine, https://www.hopkinsmedicine.org/health/healthy_heart/know_your_risks/the-heart-test-you-may-needbut-likely-havent-heard-of.

disease itself. In addition, let's be real: sugar is a booming business. Just think of all the food that's made tastier with the help of corn syrup, fructose, and other cornerstones of the processed foods industry. Sugar and its derivatives help products fly off the shelves, even though they're poisoning us in the process.

Bottom line?

If you want to avoid heart disease, forget obsessing over cholesterol. Get obsessed over the amount of excess sugar you're putting into your body and how it's putting you at risk for serious medical repercussions.

KEY TAKEAWAYS

I encounter so many people who have the passion and ambition it takes to optimize their health through their fuel intake, but the problem is that despite their determination and resilience, nutritional fallacies make optimization a challenging endeavor. But pursuing accurate information about health shouldn't be limited by corporate ulterior motives, special interests, and faulty research.

After all, this is *your* body. This is your life. The lobbyists, industries, politicians, and researchers elevating false information for their own personal gain are a tragedy.

You deserve better. It might not be fair that we've got to unlearn much of what we have been told to be true about nutrition and health, but it's just the reality.

If you want to become unstoppable, it's time to open up your mind. Avoid getting stuck in the infinite loop I found myself in in my early thirties, following the same conventional wisdom about health and nutrition, but getting nowhere. We must follow the lead of those who contributed to the creation of this chapter—people like Robb Wolf and Dr. Zoë Harcombe and many others—and reject these limiting beliefs so we can move forward in health.

Learn more about sugar from the experts at www.unstoppablebook.com/chapter7.

CHAPTER 8

THE ROLE OF EVOLUTION

Modern humans like you and me tend to treat what society has learned in the last couple hundred years as facts.

But in reality, the last two hundred years are a blip on the radar in the broad scope of human evolution.

Case in point: nearly four billion years ago, organisms appeared on planet Earth. Two million years ago, different human species began to evolve and spread throughout Africa and Eurasia. Two hundred thousand years ago, *Homo sapiens* evolved in East Africa. Around fifty thousand years ago, Neanderthals became extinct, kicking off what's known as the cognitive revolution,[38] or the time

---

38   Richard G. Klein, "Anatomy, Behavior, and Modern Human Origins," *Journal of World Prehistory* 9, no. 2 (1995): 167-198, https://www.researchgate.net/publication/227299108_Anatomy_Behavior_and_Modern_Human_Origins.

when our ancestors began to develop artifacts and create innovative techniques for hunting and gathering. Then, about thirteen thousand years ago, *Homo floresiensis* went extinct, leaving *Homo sapiens* the only remaining human species on Earth. It wasn't until twelve thousand years ago that the agricultural revolution began, five thousand years ago that religion and money appeared, and approximately five hundred years ago that the scientific revolution began.

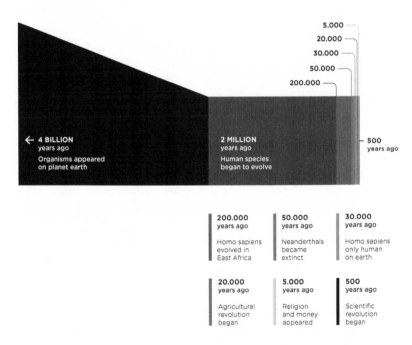

Why give a short history lesson here? To put the history of humankind into perspective. That's because while we see recent history as enough of a data set to draw conclusions from, the last couple hundred years are a blip on the radar in the broad scope of human history.

Humans are great at moving forward, adept at looking into the future, creating new things, and putting ideas into motion. But when you look at diet, nutrition, and wellness, it would be beneficial for us to look backward in time to see how we evolved. By analyzing the major events in evolutionary history, we can learn a lot about some of the problems we face today. Hopefully, in doing so, we can solve them before we, too, go extinct.

BRINGING EVOLUTION INTO THE PRESENT

Technology has changed our lives in so many ways. But nothing has changed human life more in such a short amount of time than nutrition. While some modern laboratory studies on animals (specifically rodents) are helpful, there's no data set more comprehensive than the one produced by millions of years of human evolution. By looking to the past, we can learn a lot about how to build a healthier future.

When talking about evolution, I'm referring to Darwinian evolution: the work of biologist Charles Darwin in the 1800s that highlighted how organisms change—their ability to compete, thrive, and reproduce. Many have used the phrase "survival of the fittest" to summarize one of the most important parts of his work. This notion is insightful for us today, as we explore what our species has done to not only survive but also thrive. This means understanding two things: one, that change from a biological standpoint happens extremely slowly, and two, that these changes can be both positive and negative. We want to use evolution to our advantage.

At a base, instinctive level, humans do four things: fight, flee, feed, and fornicate. I think each of these speaks to Darwin's idea of small variations over time and the ability to compete, survive, and reproduce. Our bodies are naturally inclined to do each of these things. We fight to protect. We flee if we're in danger. We feed to survive individually. We fornicate to survive communally.

So, what does human evolution tell you about optimizing your health and wellness? Answering this question means following these simple steps as part of a personal inventory:

- Notice how your body is operating, both positively and negatively.
- Make a hypothesis about what might be different with your body, or your intake, based on this time in human history.
- Evaluate how our ancestors' bodies operated in this context.

- Consider how we can accelerate evolution with unlimited access to things that our ancestors might not have had, like technology, transportation, trade, and the internet.

After taking this personal inventory of sorts, let's consider something like sugar.

Though humans have been on Earth for 2.5 million years, the agricultural revolution was only 12,000 years ago. This seems like a long time ago right now, but if all of human history were measured in a year, the agricultural boom would've began just two days ago. *Two days ago!*

So, when you take a look at something current, like our outrageous increase in consumption of sugar over the last one hundred years—a 900 percent increase—it's true that we could probably adapt to consuming copious amounts of sugar *at some point*, but it would take a few thousand years, or even hundreds of thousands of years to do.

Put simply, our bodies haven't had time to adapt to such a dramatic increase in consumption of sugar.

That's why we've seen such a meteoric rise in obesity and related chronic diseases. Millions of years ago, our ancestors were eating sugar, but not massive amounts of refined sugars. Back then, sugar came from the fruits they picked, and access to them would've been dependent upon seasonality. When we consider these fundamental differences, we can walk away with some small clues to how we should be eating today. For example, perhaps it's best to consume less sugar overall, and to eat fruit minimally, and only when in season.

As you read this, you might be thinking of a person you know who drinks two or three sodas a day, but doesn't seem to have any complications with his or her health and appears to be healthy—maybe even skinny. This is obviously confusing. But it's hard to determine if, below the surface, your friend is suffering deleterious effects of sugar consumption, such as inflammation, or is poised to encounter long-term complications down the road. While it's true that some people's bodies do handle sugar slightly better than others—after all, that's how natural selection works—I'd rather not risk those types of problems down the road, and, instead, adopt healthier practices today.

Related to the consumption of refined sugars is the consumption of carbohydrates. Although I won't go too deep into this right now, author Mark Sisson summarizes this well in his book *Primal Blueprint 21-Day Total Body Transformation* when he writes, "Our ancestors went for days without anything to eat, and carbohydrates were extremely scarce for two million years. The truth is, fat is the preferred fuel for human metabolism."

The idea is simple: learn from the evolution of our species.

In fact, looking at our evolutionary history and ancestors provides us with important hints and clues about how we should live our lives in the present day. Evolution can even provide insights about a number of areas like nutrition, diet, sleep, bowel movements, outdoor activity, sun exposure, the effect of seasons, and scheduling meals.

EVOLUTIONARY CLUES

With each passing season, your life unfolds. The sun rises and sets, and with each new day, you have the ability to align yourself with that flow, or not. But the more time I've spent researching this part of our evolutionary history, the more it's become clear to me how important adhering to these flows can be for optimal health and wellness. Our ancestors used seasons and other natural phenomena as a guide for eating, living, and a means of survival.

But today, life is very different.

Food is no longer scarce in many parts of the world. Fruit is sourced and distributed globally, and available in temperature-controlled grocery stores 365 days a year. Many people, even those of modest means, can find plentiful food, perhaps not always the healthiest, in close proximity at almost all times. This is a completely different experience from that of our ancestors.

In the book *Sapiens* by Yuval Noah Harari, the author provides us with a very interesting clue about human evolution that I find fascinating. He calls our attention to something he calls "the gorging gene," which is the idea that humans are designed to gorge on food for the sake of survival. For example, when our ancestors saw ripe fruit, they quickly ate it because nature was telling them to do so. Their consumption of food was entirely based on their relationship with the earth and the passing of the seasons. Fruit was ripe for only a limited amount of time, so they took advantage of it. Not doing so would be a waste of a valuable resource. What's more, as the book points out, your body also has a natural mechanism that partners with the seasons: it'll add fat (long-term energy storage) when you eat fruit, which makes sense, as you'll need this energy for winter.

Given the relatively short period of time that's elapsed between our ancestral way of life and today, it makes sense that our bodies haven't quite been able to get rid of this so-called gorging gene. When we see food in front of us, we want to eat it—sometimes even when we're not hungry at all.

The only problem?

As I mentioned above, food is readily available *everywhere* nowadays. From fresh, whole foods to packaged goods filled with preservatives and chemicals, it's all readily accessible, and often for very little money. And therein lies the problem: saddled with an evolutionary imperative to eat what's before us, we do exactly that. With access to all types of food, all the time, our bodies tell us to feast as if winter is coming. But it never does. And in the process, we get fat.

Although there are still hunter-gatherer societies in remote parts of the world, chances are pretty high if you're reading this book that you're not living in one. Instead, like me, you live in a world where a famine is unlikely to occur anytime soon. And that means you've got to negotiate making the right food choices in the midst of a dizzying array of options, and with an evolutionary imperative to eat. It's essentially a recipe for disaster.

Since our bodies are used to a feast-and-famine flow—the cycle of different foods growing from the earth, the lack of food during the winter, or periods when it was impossible to forage or hunt—it's important to take a clue from our ancestors and apply a similar approach in our modern lives.

We'll talk more about fasting later on, but evolutionarily speaking, it's worth exploring in our experimentation if we feel better and operate better when gorging certain natural foods, cycling those foods in and out of our diet, and then periodically fasting. Of course, this doesn't mean that these ideas will produce 100 percent optimization for your nutrition, since each person evolves differently, but it does mean that all of these ideas are worth trying because they're rooted in our past.

In addition to using evolution to inform experimentation around diet, I urge you to use it as a guide for other aspects of daily life, such as sleep and exercise. For example, history tells us that our ancestors went to sleep around sunset and got up around sunrise. Interestingly, many scientific studies have indicated that the most restorative sleep is between 9:00 p.m. and 1:00 a.m., which doesn't shift if you get to bed later—you can't make it up. If you don't sleep during those times, the benefits are just lost. We also know that nine hours or more of sleep is healthiest for humans, which all goes back to our history and how we've been programmed to survive.

Even though humans have been on Earth for 2.5 million years, the agricultural revolution was only 12,000 years ago. As I mentioned at the beginning of this section, if all of human history were measured in one year, the agricultural boom would've began just two days ago. During this relatively short period of time, humans have been confronted with large-scale changes that have made food more readily available than ever before. And although modern life is completely different from how our ancestors lived, our bodies don't know the difference. But the reality is, we're not doomed. By leveraging what we know about our ancestral past, we can experiment to find better ways of living, and healthier ways to manage environmental change.

USING EVOLUTION TO YOUR ADVANTAGE

There are some people who will argue that because of our evolutionary pasts, humans should start replicating our ancestors' way of living as much as possible. That's why some people focus so much on so-called paleo diets, living off the land, and walking around barefoot or in minimalist footwear (to replicate the feeling of going barefoot). I've nothing against this—after all, everyone's on their own journey. But rather than making a massive departure from modern living, I'm much more into the idea of using common sense to guide what we take away from our evolutionary past. Which is why when I look at what we can take away from our ancestors and apply to our modern lives, I immediately identify three areas:

1. Gorging
2. Fasting
3. Sleeping

Throughout my research into ancestral practices, this trio came up time after time. It led me to conclude that these three elements—gorging, fasting, and sleeping—are core components of what it means to be human. And, when we're able to optimize these for these three things, it goes a long way toward achieving the balance that drives true health and wellness.

But why's this so important?

Well, as I've discussed throughout the book so far, being healthy isn't easy. It's hard to stay on track, particularly when we're constantly bombarded by pseudoscience, corporate meddling, and less-than-accurate information about what it means to be healthy. By focusing on these three core elements, we not only put ourselves on the fastest track toward health, we also dramatically simplify our thinking around the topic.

So, how do you make sure you leverage the power of these three components in your life to accelerate your own optimization? Let me break it down further into three easy parts:

Marry modern resources and your own revolutionary awareness. By understanding how our ancestors lived, and what biological processes were key to their health and survival—gorging, fasting, sleeping—you can pursue similar activities, but with greater access to modern resources. Use this to your advantage. Devise tests you can run in each of the aforementioned areas and see how you feel following a similar ancestral pattern. In the area of nutrition, I've found it's also useful to identify and test the high-quality whole foods that would've sustained our ancestors long ago. For example, as evidenced by multiple books on ancestral eating patterns, carbohydrates certainly weren't available for consumption. That meant that *fat* was the fuel of choice. Today, we can find healthy forms of fat just about anywhere: scientists point out that MCT oil is a potent source of healthy fat and energy that can be added to everything from coffee to salad dressing.

Use science and research to your advantage. Here's where a critical lens is of the utmost importance. Throughout my life, I trusted pseudoscientific information about nutrition and health that, at best, wasn't accurate. At worst, it was dangerous to my health. Even though my body felt *awful* doing the things that pop-culture science prescribed, I kept doing them because I thought they were "right." This caused me to think there was something wrong with me. I internalized this, doubled down on bad practices, and ended up doing more harm than good. All of these challenges would've been avoided if I'd dug deeper into the source of my information and evaluated whether the advice was credible or not. But what I learned can save you the headaches and frustration and get you to optimal health faster.

Beware of abundance. I caution that the wealth of information and resources available to you can also be a double-edged sword. And from this abundance can come unhealthiness and disease. For example, you can purchase macadamia nuts year-round, but you can also, for the first time, order any salty, greasy restaurant food within a couple of minutes through an app on your phone. You can use science to your advantage with MCT oil, but science is also being used for your detriment. For example, in the last chapter, Robb Wolf talked about Doritos Roulette—how variation in taste makes us want to keep eating, even if we aren't hungry. Food scientists have figured out exactly how much sugar, vegetable oils, and other ingredients combine to make something that our biology responds to. It's all a trick, and they know it, and they're using it against you. Use science, research, and rigorous lines of questioning—and experimentation—to your advantage. Don't let the food and beverage industries take advantage of you.

Again, the key is to use your abundance and your privileges to your advantage—to evolve and adapt faster than evolution would typically allow. There are endless experiments you can conduct based on clues you discover about evolution, but the top three ways to use evolution to your advantage is through supplementation, cycling, and ketosis, which I'll touch on briefly here and explore more deeply in later chapters.

- *Supplementation.* This is the consumption of products that scientists or nutritionists have refined and distilled for your benefit, like a B12 or D3 dietary supplement, or something like krill oil. All of these can give you a boost to the body or the brain that's backed up by evolution, yet for the majority of human history might have only been found in foods that were in a certain region of the world. Use this to your advantage. Why wouldn't you do something simple to optimize your body and mind and take something that no one else in human history has been able to so easily consume? We didn't always have access to these nutrients, vitamins, and minerals, so, use this major area to experiment with optimization.
- *Cycling.* This is partnering with evolution in forcing your body into these natural feast-and-famine cycles through things like fasting, calorie reduction, or even things like exercising or changing your environment and sleep.
- *Ketosis.* This goes back to the idea of calorie balance and utilizing the natural energy-release mechanisms in our bodies. We've learned this through modern science and careful study of our evolutionary past.

Allow the general ideas in this chapter about our evolutionary past to pique your curiosity and pull you deeper into the journey of optimizing your health and wellness. Open your eyes to the realm of possibilities around you to access foods and nutrients that no one in the course of human history has been in a position to so readily and easily consume. Cut spending in an area of your life that isn't beneficial to your health and use that money to purchase supplements or foods that will benefit your life, body, and mind. Become aware of how wealthy and power-hungry minds in our biggest industries want to also use science and research to manipulate you and use you for your purchasing power. Go backward into human evolution to find what can be used to help you evolve and adapt faster.

What aspects of your body and mind will you tap into?

What within you has been there all along but has yet to be unleashed?

Get ready to find out.

Evolution gives us clues about what's best for our bodies. Learn more at www.unstoppablebook.com/chapter8.

CHAPTER 9

HOW DID WE GET HERE?

We spent a lot of time talking about the distant past in the last chapter, and now I want to bring us closer to the present to take a look at how economic systems, financial incentives, and ideological trends have had a major impact on how we think about health and wellness. While earlier on I talked about where the US went wrong with regard to perpetuating myths about nutrition, in this chapter, I'll focus on distilling the *systemic* problems: how science and our medical system have been influenced by pharmaceutical companies, big business, food manufacturers, and policy subsidies.

By answering the question "How did we get here?" you'll identify the underlying motives at play in our times, helping you to discover truth that's more relevant and valuable to your life.

THE PROBLEM

Where did we go wrong?

Strangely enough, many of the problems we see in the world of nutrition, science, and health start with the word we've been using in a positive way throughout this book: "optimization."

You see, a core function of capitalism is to optimize processes and people. And generally, that's a good thing. It creates jobs. It inspires new ideas and competition. It can produce financial security as wealth multiplies. But this kind of optimization can also aim to get the most out of every dollar, even if that means doing something immoral or manipulative. At its worst, it can elevate profits over people, which is what has happened in the context of health and wellness. In this context, generating more money is the goal—not evolution, not unity, not the overall health of our society.

Put simply, it's good for both big business and the pharmaceutical industry to have a needy population of overweight and unhealthy people. Without the right information about the right foods, the right exercise, or the right health practices, it's easy to feed this population the products they make. It's easy to hook them on foods designed to leave them wanting *more*. And if they ever wonder about the safety of buying and consuming what you sell, these same companies have the means to fund research that'll tell you it's okay to keep eating their chemicals, preservatives, vegetable fats, and refined sugars. To obscure wrongdoing, they may even tell you that something else is the culprit to avoid implication in a large-scale public health crisis, similar to what the sugar industry did in 1968.

In 2016, the US market made up 45 percent of the pharmaceutical industry, generating $446 billion a year selling drugs to treat complications from obesity.[39] They even made money selling drugs to treat the side effects of other drugs they had already sold to the US population and beyond. Hungry to establish recurring forms of revenue as well as new revenue streams, there are drugs for everything. That's because the pharmaceutical industry's best customer is an unhealthy one. But they've optimized their business and processes for this exact outcome. And that's how optimization is used from a greedy, capitalistic perspective. While there are certainly companies that are trying to do better, most companies are in relentless pursuit of profit.

That being said, I hope this book will allow you to see how you can put a stop to this by taking back control from these corporations and optimizing yourself using credible

---

39 "U.S. Pharmaceutical Industry—Statistics & Facts," Statista, https://www.statista.com/topics/1719/pharmaceutical-industry/.

information about health and wellness. I hope this book empowers you to dare to optimize yourself with the same rigor that they're applying to business. In this way, you give yourself far more agency than I ever gave to myself. And that gives you a clear choice: continue to follow the lead of big corporations, or forge your own path. I hope you'll choose the latter.

THE COST OF RESEARCH VERSUS THE COST OF DOING NOTHING

Scientific research costs money. Lots of money. So, when it comes to funding new studies, it has always been easy for those with a lot of it to wield enormous power in terms of which research gets funded and how the results are interpreted. As a result, up until the early 2000s, it wasn't uncommon for studies to be conducted and data to be manipulated in order to pull out a "positive" finding.

But things started to change with the passage of the FDA Modernization Act in 1997, whichrequired that academic entities register their research, along with key information about it, like "the study's purpose, recruitment status, design, eligibility criteria, locations and pre-specified primary and secondary outcomes."[40] Then, in 2001, major

---

40   Robert M. Kaplan and Veronica L. Irvin, "Likelihood of Null Effects of Large NHLBI Clinical Trials Has Increased over Time," *PLOS ONE* 10, no. 8 (2015): e0132382. https://doi.org/10.1371/journal.pone.0132382

academic journals expanded on efforts to drive transparency by requiring those who ran "randomized clinical trials"—or RCTs for short—to register their research in order to be considered for publication in major journals. The goal of these efforts was simple: require more rigor and focus around research at the outset to limit any "creative freedom" in interpreting the data after the fact to suit specific outcomes, biases, or corporate agendas.

About fifteen years later in 2015, in a report on the impact of these changes,[41] public policy experts and the scientific community delivered some surprising news: research that took place *after* the changes in the early 2000s yielded fewer positive results. That is to say that more often than not, the research and experiments didn't yield as many clear, specific outcomes compared with those in the past.[42]

Coincidence? Maybe. But probably not.

What the strict guidelines around research had done was enforce a vetting mechanism that would help differentiate credible research from the kind that might've been manipulated in order to produce a certain finding or nar-

41   Ibid.

42   Kevin Drum, "Chart of the Decade: Why You Shouldn't Trust Every Scientific Study You
     See," *Mother Jones*, November 8, 2018, https://www.motherjones.com/kevin-drum/2018/11/
     chart-of-the-decade-why-you-shouldnt-trust-every-scientific-study-you-see/.

rative. It would, essentially, allow research to do what it's designed to do: help people make discoveries. Ultimately, it forced the scientific community to police itself, and, in the process, squeeze out those who would be inclined to manipulate the data for a desired outcome.

To visualize the shift more easily, check out the scatterplot. As you can see, in the decades leading up to RCT reform in the early 2000s, there were numerous studies that yielded positive outcomes. But after the year 2000, when scrutiny around research increased, most studies yielded null effects, or *no outcome one way or the other*. For anyone interpreting this data, it can't be ignored that around the same time as scrutiny around RCTs increased, the number of studies with positive outcomes decreased.[43]

---

43   Kaplan and Irvin, "Likelihood of Null Effects."

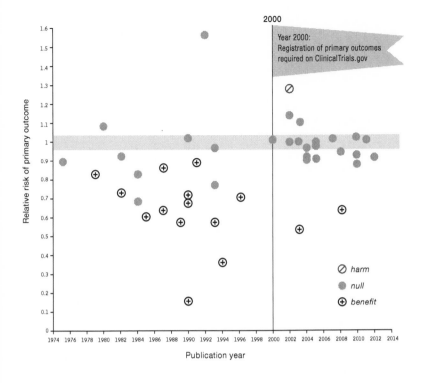

Let's be clear: the culture of research is brutal, and the pressure not to waste funding on data that doesn't yield a powerful narrative is real. What's more, if you're a scientist who's interested in potentially challenging long-held beliefs around fat and sugar, and their impact on health and wellness, it's going to be difficult to find the funding and support you need. But it's important work that must be done to dispel the myths surrounding major health problems and halt the growth of chronic disease in the US and around the world. Soon, the cost of conducting this kind of research will pale in comparison to the rising cost of medicine to address these issues.

In fact, the numbers around chronic disease in the US provide a clear—but alarming—narrative about the current health of Americans. According to recent research:[44]

- Approximately 45 percent of all Americans have a chronic disease, and the number continues to grow.
- More than two-thirds of all deaths are caused by one or more of the following chronic diseases: heart disease, cancer, stroke, chronic obstructive pulmonary disease, and diabetes.
- Chronic diseases are to blame for 70 percent of deaths in the US.

In a nation with some of the best healthcare in the world, how does this happen? How do we reconcile having access to leading technology and medical treatments, yet 70 percent of deaths are due to chronic disease?

To find an answer, one need not look any further than how a great deal of the medical establishment operates. Instead of an improve-and-maintain approach, modern medicine has been artfully constructed around a break-and-fix model. That is to say that we're really great at solving short-term problems, but not anywhere near as efficient at managing long-term care and patient out-

---

44 Wullianallur Raghupathi and Viju Raghupathi, "An Empirical Study of Chronic Diseases in the United States: A Visual Analytics Approach to Public Health," *International Journal of Environmental Research and Public Health* 15, no. 3 (2018): 431, https://www.ncbi.nlm.nih.gov/pmc/articles/PMC5876976/.

comes. The illness that can't be solved by giving someone a pill each day goes wildly mismanaged as patients are sent off with very little guidance or follow-up regarding chronic conditions. Rarely do doctors discuss diet, nutrition, and the underlying cause of chronic disease to improve patient outcomes. And how could they? With an ever-increasing roster of patients, the most they can do is have a quick conversation and send people off with a prescription.

The trouble is, people still need answers. People want a better way. They don't want to succumb to chronic disease and become a burden on family and friends—they want to lead better, more fulfilling lives instead of fearing for the future.

The overarching goal of modern medicine today, as I see it, is to manage symptoms at a reasonable and productive level so people don't complain, and feel better in the short-term, especially as people get older. Instead of examining the symptoms, we mask and manage them. But, as is often the case, this creates new issues, drug interactions, and a lower quality of life. That's why, after years of research, and my own very bumpy journey to health and wellness, I've made the following conclusion: we must take our health into our own hands.

WEIGHING THE SCIENCE

You and I—we're lucky. Today, thanks to the internet, we've got the privilege of instant access to tons of data and source material from people who are far more intelligent than we'll ever be. And, despite what's happened in the past, the realm of science is still an incredible area to gather ideas for personal experimentation. The challenge is finding the right science—that is, the kind that's rigorous and comprehensive. But once you do, instead of moving *against* evolutionary history, you can evolve faster, using the wealth of resources and information out there to your own benefit. And I want to support you in your effort to do just that.

But before you can dig into the research that'll help guide you on your journey, it's good to develop a critical lens for evaluating the material you'll come across, as well as a solid understanding of the types of research out there. That's why I have three simple things for you to remember:

Don't believe the hype. We live in a headline-driven world. Whether we're on our phones or watching television, commuting to work or spending time with family, we're constantly barraged by media that demands our attention. And, since news cycles move fast, flashy headlines have become the norm. I realize what I'm about to say might seem like a silly example, but it proves my point, so humor me. Say the headline of a study says, "Jump off a building if you want to live longer." Absurd, right? As strange as it is, this might not be a completely inaccurate headline if there was *one* person in the study who jumped off of a building, somehow survived, and out of that transformative near-death experience, went on to live a long and healthy life. Of course, if you expanded your data set of people who jumped off buildings over a period of time, you'd most likely find that the majority of those individuals died. Yet the headline focused on the *one* person who survived, in order to catch people's attention. These days, in a world that optimizes for clicks, headlines like these are the norm, and they're incredibly misleading.

Know your source(s). Today, content—"reports," blog posts, sponsored content—is king. For big companies, it's the foundation of both paid and organic advertising, as well as clicks and ad impressions. And while that's been great for search marketing and related industries, the changing nature of content has made it much harder to distinguish high-quality, impartial material from content that's created to advance a brand or corporate agenda. So, the next time you're wondering about the credibility of the health and wellness content you're reading, take a look at where the information came from—an academic institution or a brand? A well-respected medical journal or an industry publication trying to make its info sound more trustworthy? Evaluate sources and ask yourself what those behind them stand to gain by advancing specific narratives.

Be your own investigative journalist. Besides sidestepping the hype and finding reputable sources, it's imperative that you become your own investigative journalist during this process. When you come across compelling info, dig deeper into how the data was collected, and under what circumstances. If it's large-scale research, check out who the participants were, and how the results were analyzed. Do you detect whether or not there's bias in the tone of the write-up of the findings? It might be a bit dry at first, but you should actually read the studies you come across. I know it's not the most entertaining reading, but you're literally reading for your own good, so you owe it to yourself.

That being said, studies are still incredible sources for possible ideas for experimentation, inspiration, and information, just *not* absolute truths. Your job is to absorb the information, compare it to our evolutionary history, and make decisions about what works best for you. Typically, you'll do this through many different types of studies: epidemiological, single-blind, double-blind, and control group. I'll outline each briefly now:

- *Epidemiological study.* This type of study involves large, diverse samples that are intended to reflect a greater whole. While sizable in nature, these types of studies can be useful in assessing the breadth of certain phenomena, but not necessarily depth. In most cases, these types of studies will be useful starting points, but don't mistake breadth of research for conclusiveness of findings.

- *Single-blind study.* A single-blind study involves two groups of participants: the intervention group and the control group. While study participants don't know which group they're in, researchers do. Typically, single-blind studies are used to test the efficacy of medications.

- *Double-blind study.* A double-blind study is the gold standard of studies because it's the most expensive and the most difficult to execute. In these types of studies, the researcher who's conducting the study and managing the groups doesn't know who is in what group. In the total absence of potential bias, this kind of study ensures greater accuracy.

- *Control group.* Studies that use a control group are probably the most widely used in health and diet research because they're cheaper than conducting a single-blind study or double-blind study, and they're still fairly accurate. Control groups and experimental groups are treated the same throughout an experiment, except for interventions made by researchers on the experimental group.

Although each of these different types of studies is very valuable, you probably understand from previous chapters that no single study is flawless. Scientists are brilliant people, but also humans who possess biases, just like everyone else. So, recognize that no single body of research is the absolute truth—and that's okay. The beauty of science is the potential for *discovery*, and that's what all good research should yield.

Remember, the framework is all about being tuned into *your* feedback. You're not trying to prove or disprove whether something works for a massive group of respondents in an epidemiological study—you're trying to uncover how something works for *you*. Say, for example, you come across a study that talks about the importance of lowering your cholesterol. The next step would be for you to find anything that you can regarding the underlying factors, funding, or potential motives behind the study. Who conducted it? What might their possible motive be in conducting this kind of research? What kind of study was it? If you decide that the study is credible to you and worth trying to replicate in order to lower your cholesterol, then do it. If your cholesterol is lowered and you feel better, awesome. It means you learned something about yourself that you can trust, and also happens to be rooted in credible research. Your own output is all that matters.

BUILDING YOUR MEDICAL DREAM TEAM

Medicine is a field of study. But medicine is also a *business*. And that means it's subject to the same types of optimizations you'd see in typical business environments. Doctors, like many other professions, are pressured by insurance companies—the people who pay their bills—to see more patients in less time, and provide more positive short-term outcomes than negative ones. When you go to the doctor's office today, chances are you'll see your doctor for only five minutes or so before he or she rushes off to see the next patient in line.

Let's be real: there's no way for one person to get to know another in five minutes or less.

And, there's definitely *no* way that a doctor in this kind of environment has the time to provide you with the kind of comprehensive, personalized care you need. More often than not, patients like you and me leave with a pill, and a lot of unanswered questions. To put it simply, the system is broken.

So, how'd we find ourselves in this mess?

Simple: our entire medical system is built around sickness, not health. Most people only go to the doctor when something is wrong. When disaster strikes, we have some of the best care in the world to fix what's broken. But when it comes to long-term health and wellness, there's little education or support for patients. This "break-and-fix" mentality is very different from one that's focused on improving and maintaining.

Let me ask you a question—if you had a complicated year with your finances, and it was tax season, would you want an amazing accountant who could help put you in the best financial position possible? Or would you want one that's just...okay? You'd obviously want the one who's amazing. What about if you had the option of sending your kid to a top-rated school with an outstanding educational program, or one with mediocre teachers and no focus on academic achievement? You'd choose the top-rated school, I'd imagine. And in any similar scenario, the majority of people would choose the option that delivers an optimal outcome.

So, why is it, when it comes to medical care, we don't apply the same reasoning? Why is it that, instead of looking for medical treatment that gets us closer to optimal health and wellness, we settle for just "okay"?

I've spent a lot of time thinking about why this is. To find an answer, I looked back to how I managed my own health in my twenties. Instead of seeking optimal medical care, I accepted the bare minimum my doctors could give, which consisted of an annual physical and a blood panel, and usually, that was it. If there was nothing glaring in the reports that came back, I usually didn't think about it again for another year.

I've noticed that, for some reason, we usually just accept what doctors tell us without pushing back, even if things seem wrong. Throughout my research into health and wellness over the last few years, I've decided this is wrong. We need to take responsibility for our bodies, and put ourselves in the driver's seat when it comes to our medical care. I've had to put this into practice recently, too: my girlfriend, Dawn, has ulcerative colitis (UC), so we went and saw the top specialist in the world in Los Angeles to experiment with a new test that many who are on the frontlines of UC and Crohn's research are raving about. We paid $300, had the test performed—a noninvasive monitoring technique that detects inflammation in the gut—and it was incredibly insightful. It was eye-opening and extremely encouraging to Dawn. The specialist recommended that she continue the test when we returned home to Las Vegas. But when she went to her specialist in Las Vegas, the doctor told Dawn that he'd never heard of the test and wouldn't be able to run it. Although we were surprised, we pushed back and essentially told him, "We don't care if you don't do it for other people or have never heard of it. That's not what we asked you. We're telling you that the top specialist in the country says that it needs to be done, so figure out a way to run the test."

I know this sounds harsh, but it's exactly what you would say to a cook at a restaurant if he said that he wasn't in the mood to cook, or to a bank teller who couldn't be bothered to help you with a transaction. You can and *should* question your doctor. It's *your* health and you're paying for it, after all. A good doctor will understand why you're doing it, and empower you with the right information. And if they don't, you can always find a new one. I've done it plenty of times. So build your team.

Building your medical team takes effort, just like everything else. But the results—attention, personalized care, access to new modes of care, and ultimately, better health—will be the reward. This is what it takes to go beyond average and experience optimal health.

To set expectations, though, let me be clear: all these things won't be found in a single provider. It'll require you to do research and find the different specialists for what you're testing and questions you have. But in taking ownership of your journey and doing the extra work to assemble your medical dream team, you'll position yourself to get the most out of the brilliant minds around you, and evolve in a way that very few people can.

Ready to get started building your medical dream team? Let's quickly review the types of doctors and areas of specialty you may want to identify and include:

- *Concierge medicine.* A concierge doctor has very different incentives than most doctors. He or she will usually charge you a monthly or annual fee. Concierge doctors spend more time with their patients and focus more on long-term outcomes rather than short-term outcomes. They're still focused on traditional medicine for the most part and will write prescriptions as a solution, but in general, you're paying to get more of their time, greater access to them as a resource, and the ability to go deeper into areas of concern for you. Unlike traditional doctors, concierge doctors have a fixed number of patients and a fixed amount of money coming in each month. Having fewer patients means they can obviously spend more time with each one. Their business model is different. Insurance doesn't pay, and they don't charge insurance in order to reduce their overhead billing. That's why this type of doctor usually also has a higher cost—anywhere from $1,000 to $10,000 a year, depending on the doctor. But concierge doctors are becoming more popular. A growing subset of doctors follow a hybrid model called "direct primary care." They accept insurance and still deal with the larger numbers of patients, but place more emphasis on achieving long-term goals.
- *Functional medicine.* Functional doctors often serve as a solid foundation for building your medical dream team. Although they're similar to concierge doctors and usually bill monthly or annually, functional

doctors usually take a much more future-oriented approach to your health by proactively ordering tests and looking for ways to optimize your current and long-term health. When you look for a functional doctor, don't settle—you really need someone who wants to work alongside you as you experiment, and provide valuable guidance along the way. From there, you can add a nutrition expert or a cardiologist or other specialists who can help you with something specific.

- *Primal doctors.* Primal doctors are similar to functional doctors but have areas of specialized focus. In my experience, they're more focused on the paleo lifestyle, with a tight emphasis on diet, consumption, and lifestyle.
- *Online medicine and telemedicine.* This is an area that's emerging, and I find it very interesting, mostly because I think everyone should have access to great doctors and healthcare. Online and telemedicine make that a possibility. With either, you can use an app or a website to have a video chat with your doctors, no matter where you are.

Assembling your medical dream team is about finding people who are qualified and prepared to support you on your journey to becoming unstoppable. This means you've got to find individuals who believe in and understand why you're leveraging this framework, and will be there to answer your questions along the way. That being said, some people are lucky enough to already have physicians who are open to this approach. If you're one of the few who do, assembling your dream team may require less effort. Regardless, as you're kicking off this process, it's helpful to ask yourself if your physician will be open to collaborating with you as you run experiments within the framework. If you don't think he or she will be, that may be a sign you need to look for someone else. Again, you need people who will empower you with credible info and support throughout what will no doubt be a long journey.

Building your own medical dream team is about taking ownership and not waiting for someone else to fix your problems. Don't be discouraged if it takes you a few tries to assemble the right people to support you throughout this process. In my experience, it's never as easy as looking someone up and hitting it off immediately. It's an investment of time, but in the end, it's absolutely worth it.

Now that we've covered the framework, common myths, and how we got here, let's dig into the practical stuff so that you can begin experimenting and optimizing your life.

**Get tips and advice for assembling
your medical dream team at
www.unstoppablebook.com/chapter9.**

PART III

—

EXPERIMENTS

CHAPTER 10

FUEL YOURSELF: THE UNSTOPPABLE LIFESTYLE I

If you put diesel in a car that takes gasoline, or gasoline in a truck that takes diesel, neither vehicle will operate normally. In fact, a mechanic would tell you to tow both cars to a shop so that the problematic fuel could be flushed out. If you decided to disregard the mechanic and continue driving with the wrong fuel, you'd ultimately cause short- and long-term damage to both cars. Curiously, this isn't unlike what happens to the human body when we continually give it the wrong fuel: it may run for a short time, but ultimately, there are some serious repercussions, like chronic illness, weight gain, brain fog, lethargy, and more.

Despite this, few Americans critically examine the

food they put into their own bodies each day. Instead of treating meals as an opportunity to fuel ourselves from a nutritional perspective, we often—knowingly or unknowingly—consume preservative-filled snacks and high-carbohydrate processed foods that our bodies didn't evolve to process. In my twenties, even once I became aware of the fact that some foods were healthier than others, I still didn't really understand that the *type* and *quality* of food that I was putting in my body was having a direct impact on my energy levels, metabolism, and overall well-being. To add insult to injury, I believed for quite some time that all the perils of eating the wrong foods could be offset by rigorous and even obsessive exercise. Looking back now, I see how reckless this behavior was, and understand why I struggled so much with my weight and energy levels over the years: I wasn't fueling my body the right way.

When my children were born, I made a vow not to treat their diets with this kind of recklessness. Based on thorough research and a lot of learning, Dawn and I had a good understanding of what they needed fuel-wise each step of the way. So we began to view food strictly as a means of fuel for our children's growth. The more we could provide the right foods at each stage of development, as well as educate them about making smart choices, the greater the likelihood they'd reach their maximum potential. It's something every parent strives to do.

After watching my kids grow and thrive with the right foods, it struck me as odd that, as adults, we suddenly stop viewing food as fuel for optimal wellness. It got me thinking: what would our bodies look like if we, as adults, treated our food intake as vital to our continued development? What would our world look like if we stopped to consider the ways in which our current obsession with processed foods contributed to myriad chronic illnesses and rising levels of obesity? These were important questions I felt compelled to answer. But before I could answer any of these questions, I had to explore my own relationship with food.

Like many Americans, I'd never treated food as *fuel*. I often made poor decisions about what I put in my body, and as a busy person, I was often eating on the go. In fact, even when I *wasn't* busy, I was in a hurry, as if I were in a speed-eating competition with only myself. It was pretty ludicrous.

But where had I gone wrong?

The yoga teacher training I started shortly after moving to Las Vegas provided some clues. There was one component that I found specifically useful in addressing my relationship to food, and that was the practice of mindful eating. My training taught me that meals and my consumption of food were experiences to be relished, to be savored. Instead of inhaling food at breakfast, lunch, or dinner, eating mindfully meant I ate slowly, gratefully, and highly aware of each bite. This practice had an unintended effect: it forced me to consider whether or not the food I was eating would help or hurt my body. By forcing me to slow down, the practice of mindful eating gave me a higher-level awareness of what I chose to put in my body. For the kid who was always hungry growing up, who later became the adult who loved to eat, it was truly a magical moment when, after a few weeks of mindful eating, I could leave the dinner table feeling sated.

THIS ISN'T A DIET BOOK

I hate diet books. I've read far too many, and it's never gone very well.

That's why I want to be clear that what follows isn't a rigid set of rules about what you should eat. Instead, it's a set of recommendations about nutrition that I encourage you to experiment with in order to optimize your life. Think of it as a starting point, not a destination.

For me, learning to treat food as fuel was the turning point that revolutionized what and how I ate. It made me more mindful of what I was putting in my body, improved my ability to concentrate throughout the day, and gave me more energy. While everyone's body is different, I'm confident that in tandem with rigorous experimentation within the framework, this high-level approach to food and nutrition will help you take the first step toward becoming unstoppable in every facet of your life.

Throughout your experimentation with nutrition, I encourage you to keep regular logs of your experiments if you can. This will, of course, help you analyze and record key discoveries along the way. Nothing crazy—just start small, with an entry for each day in a document you can access anywhere. I suggest noting:

- When you eat
- What you eat
- How you're feeling overall:
    - Hungry?
    - Less/more frequent trips to the bathroom?
    - Any bloating or intestinal discomfort?
    - Did a meal cause you to feel unusual in some way—extra full, lethargic, etc.?

These days, it's socially acceptable to be tinkering with your diet, trying new things, and learning about your body. It's also an area that, with commitment, will allow you to see some short-term results. But I urge you to stay focused on using these nutrition experiments to identify the cause of the issue, not manage or mask the symptom. For example, a lot of times when people feel tired, they eat sugar or drink more caffeine to get a quick jolt of energy. With my framework, I'll challenge you to get to the root cause of why you feel that way and take steps to fix it. It might not yield a quick fix, but your progress toward a better *solution* gets you further in the long-term than medicating, caffeinating, or eating ever could. Be patient. Keep experimenting.

Last note about the information that follows: all the ideas I discuss in this chapter derive from both research that I respect, as well as my own personal experimentation. I'm sharing these general guidelines not to convince you of a particular diet, but to give you ideas for your own experimentation. Ultimately, I hope you find a way of eating that works for you. It doesn't matter what the best-selling nutrition books say, what the latest food fad is—it only matters how *you* feel and perform. That's it. Don't let anyone tell you otherwise. But for most of the population, these rules will work far better than the current dietary recommendations that are killing us.

Before I get into the "rules," a quick caveat: you don't have to be dogmatic about these. If you're at a social function or out with friends or with your family during a holiday or whatever it may be, enjoy yourself. These are just high-level guidelines that if you mostly follow, you'll see major results. Enjoy life!

AVOID PROCESSED SUGAR

Don't consume something if it's sweet. Sugar is a toxin, just like alcohol. The problem with the way your body processes sugar is that it's turned directly into fat, and then stored in the body. Your body is listening to what you put into it. Remember that for thousands of years fruits have signaled to your body to store the sugar for energy and turn it into fat so that you don't die during the winter. It's for a good reason that your body does that. Because of this, I avoid fruit for the most part. And I never eat refined sugars. I'll occasionally have some local honey because it's good for reducing allergies. I'll occasionally eat some blackberries, raspberries, and especially blueberries—as these are really good for you—but the thing to avoid at all costs is processed sugar, especially high-fructose corn syrup. This is horrible for you.

AVOID PROCESSED FOODS

As much as possible, stay away from anything that comes in plastic packaging. There are obviously exceptions to this, like nuts, for example, which are generally great for you. But most everything that comes in a plastic package is to be avoided, since most of what's inside is heavily processed and rife with a deadly combination of unnatural vegetable oils, sugars, and chemicals.

EAT WHOLE FOODS

Eat foods that are as close to their original state as possible. And, whenever possible, whether it's meat, a vegetable, or on rare occasions, a fruit, eat as much of it as you can. For example, when our ancestors ate bison, they ate *all of it*—the meat, the fat, the organs. That might not be as realistic these days, but to get the nutritional value, the whole entity should be considered nutrition. The same goes for fruit when you have it—if you have an apple, eat the skin, too. If you add garlic to your meals, don't use powder—which is packed with preservatives and additives—use a few whole cloves of the real thing.

Apply this guideline to your shopping, too. When I purchase my groceries, I try to buy goods that are as close to their original state as possible. Plastic packaging, again, usually means there are preservatives of some sort designed to make the food last longer than it should. Generally speaking, stay away from all the center aisles at the grocery store. Most supermarkets have all the fruits and veggies on the left or right, meat along the back, and all the processed crap in the middle.

AVOID REFINED CARBOHYDRATES

Refined carbohydrates are grain products that have been processed by a food manufacturer. Things like flour, rice, pasta, corn, and grains of all types. My general rule is that

I don't consume carbohydrates unless they're coming from green leafy vegetables. While I advise you to avoid carbohydrates, similar to the once popular Atkins diet, this doesn't mean eating a steady diet of meat—it means adding as much green to your diet as possible, and avoiding foods that are white, were white, or could be white. The only exception to this is cauliflower, which is off-white and great for you.

AVOID FRIED FOODS

Fried foods are tremendously hard on your body. The process of frying creates horrible breakdowns and bonds in the food that then create inflammation in your body. And inflammation is to be avoided at all costs. In fact, I try to limit the amount of foods in my life that cause inflammation—and fried food is one of them. The thing about fried food, too, is that most things are fried with flour or breading. It's hard to find a fried food that isn't. Also, in most, if not all, commercial frying applications like restaurants, they use vegetable oils, which create even more problematic breakdowns. So, just by eating something fried usually means that you're breaking several of these guidelines at once. There is a case to be made that certain foods fried or cooked in natural and stable fats might be okay, but again, let's keep things simple.

When I stopped eating fried foods, I could immediately

tell how much better I felt. It was like a weight had been lifted, both physically and mentally. Just think back to how you feel after you consume something fried and the temporary sensations have passed. It's hardly ever a good feeling.

EAT HEALTHY FATS

Healthy fats are usually low-protein sources (and not just oils) that are solid at room temperature—things like butter, ghee, lard, olive oil (not to be heated or cooked with, which I'll discuss more later), avocado oil, suet, avocados, cheese, and eggs. You've probably removed a lot of stuff like this from your kitchen at some point because you were told they were unhealthy. Most people, somewhere along the way, replaced these good oils with deadly vegetable oils—oils that are ultimately killing us. Your body *needs* saturated fats, but they should come from animal sources (other than avocados and some nuts).

Let's talk about oils a bit more. Chances are, you most likely need to consume more omega-3 oils, which aid in the reduction of inflammation and a host of other bodily functions. You can get omega-3 oils from foods like fish, healthy nuts, or avocado, but hydrogenated oils (the worst of all oils), vegetable oils, and omega-6 oils should be avoided at all costs.

Think I'm being crazy? Let me ask you: When was the last time you saw an oil come out of a vegetable? *Never.*

What that means is that vegetable oil itself is a creation—the result of clever manipulation, a tremendous amount of chemicals, and a lot of processing. In other words, there's nothing natural about vegetable oil. But because of a number of prevalent myths, misleading research, and special interests, the public thinks these oils are healthy. In reality, they're merely cheap goods that unfortunately have found their way into endless restaurant dishes, and countless people's pantries. Though I still eat out sometimes, I do so knowing that I'm probably consuming more vegetable oils because they're cheap, and widely used by restaurants to save money. Just be aware of this reality.

Don't worry, though, there *are* lots of healthy fats that are solid at room temperature. Eggs are an amazing source of healthy fat, though many people have been scared of eggs because they're high in cholesterol. As I've mentioned many times, the cholesterol myth is exactly that—not real. In addition, there are a lot of great paleo items that are high in healthy fats—foods that are polyunsaturated, like olives or avocados. Other sources of healthy fats are nuts, seeds, cheese (the harder, the better), coconut oil, butter, whole milk, meat, and MCT. If your diet is lacking in healthy fats, an easy way to include them is to put butter or olive oil on top of what you're already eating.

EAT LOTS OF GREEN VEGETABLES

All vegetables are great for you, so eat lots of them. The rule is simple: eat any vegetable you want. Just know that corn and ketchup are absolutely *not* vegetables, even though the US government tells our kids that they are. Generally speaking, the more color in your diet, the better. Whether it's broccoli, cauliflower, bell peppers, asparagus, rhubarb, onions, radishes, or Brussels sprouts, they're all great for you. Eat lots of them and eat lots of other leafy greens like Swiss chard, spinach, and kale. Know that lettuce has almost no redeeming value whatsoever. You can still eat it if you want, but be sure to top it with healthy fats or nontraditional salad dressing. The great thing about vegetables is that they sometimes have carbohydrate content, but most importantly, they've got fiber, which works to clean out and reset your body. It also has enzymes that help you to digest other things.

EAT FOODS THAT ARE IN SEASON

It's great that we live in a time when many of us can buy almost whatever food item we want. But this is a double-edged sword: on the one hand, with greater access to just about anything, you can easily find the healthiest items and incorporate them into your diet. For example, I love that I can buy avocados that haven't been sprayed with preservatives year-round. But, on the other hand, this wide availability of products means that sometimes, your food comes from unusual sources—and that leaves a lot of room for less-than-healthy farming techniques and nonstandard practices for fruits, vegetables, and fish. But buying foods that are in season eliminates the risk that comes from an unusual farming source, whether fruits, vegetables, or fish. Buying foods in season also means they're fresher. And if you can purchase foods from local sources, do it. We'll talk more about food quality later on, but if you buy foods that are mostly in season, you also get a natural mix of foods over time, and variation not only tastes good but is also healthier for the body.

EAT FRUITS SPARINGLY OR ELIMINATE THEM ALTOGETHER

Humans were never meant to consume multiple servings of fruit per day. Our ancestors rarely consumed fruit, and when they did, it sent a chemical signal to the body to store any excess sugar as fat so they could survive long periods without food. The idea that fruit is good for you, though, is a myth perpetuated by the Food Pyramid. Fruit should be eaten sparingly and only when it's in season, just like our ancestors did.

ENJOY COFFEE SPARINGLY AND AVOID ALCOHOL

The two biggest questions I always receive about diet and nutrition have to do with coffee and alcohol. Over half of Americans drink a cup of coffee a day and a little less than half are considered regular alcohol users. So, I have some good news and some bad news. The good news is that coffee and tea are a perfectly fine source of caffeine. The only danger to coffee is caffeine addiction, though this isn't an addiction that's going to hurt you long-term, like tobacco or alcohol. Just take a break from coffee every once in a while, especially if you are drinking multiple cups of coffee a day.

The bad news, however, is that you should avoid alcohol. It's most likely pretty damaging to the body. No one disagrees with the fact that it's a toxin. If you enjoy alcohol and just want to consume it every now and then, sure, do it, but just be clear on this: there's no benefit to drinking alcohol. And if, or when, you do consume it, moderation is necessary. There are all kinds of studies out there suggesting that drinking alcohol, specifically wine, can extend your life, but these studies are inconsistent. It's just not worth the risk. There's nothing about alcohol that falls into the optimization category. If you want to read more about these two topics, there is a bonus chapter available online through the book's website.

For more on this topic, check out the bonus chapter 4: Coffee and Alcohol, available at www.unstoppablebook.com/bonus.

KEY TAKEAWAYS

If you follow these principles most of the time, you'll optimize your body. These are principles that anyone can apply to their life or their diet and potentially see significant benefits. Follow them, and you'll feel better than you ever have before. What you'll find is that this type of diet will position your body to do two essential things: prevent insulin resistance, the catalyst for Type 2 diabetes, obesity, and cardiovascular disease; and dramatically reduce inflammation, which causes a host of ailments.

**You'll find more in-depth information
on the topics featured in this chapter at
www.unstoppablebook.com/chapter10.**

CHAPTER 11

THE UNSTOPPABLE LIFESTYLE II

Over time, the deeper I explored areas of diet and nutrition, the more fun it became. Experimenting with a low-carb, high-fat diet was my breakthrough moment, but after that, a world of experimentation opened up for me. I began looking at food quality and cooking methods, along with a host of other things. My entire mindset shifted. Everything that I put into my body became an opportunity for fuel optimization. It was then that I began to understand what it actually meant to feel unstoppable.

Instead of beating my body to a pulp through endurance sports just so that I could eat whatever I wanted, I began approaching my nutrition with the same care and concern I'd applied to managing my children's health. I began to look at everything that I purchased at the store and everything that I ate throughout the day. I began to treat my body as if it was the best gift I'd ever received—my most prized possession, and my greatest asset. I began to realize that each day I could either help my body get better or make choices that would cause it to decline faster. Every decision was an opportunity. And although that sounds like a lot of pressure, it wasn't. It was the perfect convergence of my research, experimentation, and results.

Throughout this book, I've intentionally avoided pushing readers toward a specific diet, since I recognize that everyone's body is different. But you should know that the next set of guidelines in the Unstoppable Lifestyle are built upon a modified ketogenic diet—a low-carb, high-fat diet that, in reducing carbohydrate intake, puts your body in a metabolic state of ketosis most of the time. This diet prioritizes fat for energy and eliminates all refined carbs and sugars. The key is to eat foods that are high-fat, but *not* high in protein.

Most of these suggestions, however, will also be applicable to other legitimate diets like paleo, plant-based, and others. Like the last chapter, all of these are rooted in science, research, and personal experimentation, but because these are more specific, there's more of a chance that some of these might not work for you. I just want to share what's worked well for me so that you can experiment with these ideas within the framework.

In the previous chapter, you learned the basics about nutrition as it relates to the Unstoppable Lifestyle. In the pages that follow, we'll build on that knowledge with more specific guidelines about how to optimize your fuel intake. Then we'll dig into overall food quality guidelines and continue to talk through how these changes benefit your body and mind in ways you never imagined.

LIMIT YOUR CARBS TO TEN TO FIFTY GRAMS A DAY

Monitor your intake of carbohydrates as you start experimenting with this second set of guidelines. If possible, set a baseline for how many carbs you were consuming at the beginning of your journey so you can compare and contrast how you feel once you begin to restrict intake. The goal with limiting your carbs to ten to fifty grams per day is to begin to understand under what conditions—and with what fuel—your body performs the best. If you want to ease into this process, experiment with limiting at ten-gram intervals (any length you want). This will make it easier to monitor and track the changes you feel physiologically as you further restrict carb intake. Here's a quick example of phasing in the reduction of carbs using weekly intervals, but by no means are you limited to this amount of time—make it two weeks, a month, or longer, if you want:

- Week 1—Restrict to fifty grams of carbs
- Week 2—Restrict to forty grams
- Week 3—Restrict to thirty grams
- Week 4—Restrict to twenty grams
- Week 5—Restrict to ten grams

Phased reduction of carbs makes it easier to track and manage the changes you'll see in your body. It'll also become easier to identify portion sizes and become more cognizant of what kind of carbs you want to include as part of that gram total per day. For example, the difference in my body when I "spend" a large portion of my daily carb intake on white rice feels vastly different than when I choose to eat vegetables with trace amounts of carbs and perhaps a small amount of fruit. As you start to investigate the carb counts in the foods you eat and make decisions about what will be a part of your diet at each phase, you'll become far more adept at identifying the carbs that provide more bang for your buck, so to speak. Worth noting: there's been a lot of talk lately about the role of sweet potatoes in low-carb diets like the one I follow. Although some people swear by them, I find that I'd rather keep it simple and avoid them altogether.

Things can get confusing once you open the floodgates

to all these different exceptions. I prefer to keep these guidelines crystal clear.

LIMIT YOUR PROTEIN CONSUMPTION

Our culture is obsessed with protein. You've probably heard that it's good for building muscle and that you'll waste away without it. These are myths. Neither is true. In all actuality, we, as a culture, consume *way too much* protein. Part of it is because we've never been educated about portion sizes. People tend to think that a serving of protein is an enormous steak, but it's not. Take the time to learn about portion sizes and you'll do yourself a world of good. On a high-fat diet, you'll realize that you don't need much.

EAT FAT, FAT, AND MORE FAT

It's important to consume lots of fat, since this is your body's main source of energy within this approach. And I'm not just talking about *animal* fats—I'm talking about coconut, butter, ghee, and olive oil, too. Add these fats to everything you can. For example, it's easy to incorporate fat into vegetable dishes, salads, and if you drink it, coffee. Huge slabs of steak and bacon aren't the only way to get your fat, and although you're more than welcome to do so, this is a misconception of many who follow a high-fat, low-carb diet. Eat foods like coconut, butter, ghee, and olive oil. Add these things to everything you can. You can occasionally eat lean meats like white meat with the skin on, but I urge you to choose dark meat instead, which is considered "whole" and a better choice overall. Again, this is particular, but never eat lean meats, meats without skin, or chicken breasts. Avoid pure protein.

EAT UNLIMITED VEGETABLES

The biggest misconception perpetuated by diets like Atkins, paleo, and keto is that people think that these diets are only for carnivores. That's totally not true. In fact, quite the opposite—and that's why I tell people to eat as many vegetables as you want alongside lots of fat. That's because vegetables are an extremely beneficial source of fiber, which does all sorts of amazing things like make you feel fuller for longer, keep you regular, and help to flush toxins out of your body. Although fiber can be found in grains and cereals, these are always loaded with sugar and are completely unhealthy. Just get your fiber from vegetables.

AVOID REFINED SUGARS, CARBS, FLOURS, AND GRAINS

This is a simple rule, and there's no need to draw this out: avoid everything in the list above. And, yes, for those of you who are following a paleo diet, that includes coconut sugar. Also, avoid corn, soy, and gluten. If you really want to treat yourself to something, go for it—enjoy life! But just make the conscious decision and know that you're in control.

EAT NUTS, AVOCADOS, AND HEALTHY OILS

Again, open your mind to eating other foods for fat besides animal products. Avocados are truly one of the most amazing things that you can eat on a diet like this, and they can be consumed with almost anything. It's one of the only foods that I consume consistently year-round. Adding foods like avocados to most of my meals has led to those magical moments of not feeling hungry. When it comes to consuming nuts, I recommend macadamia, almond, coconut, and walnuts. Avoid peanuts—which are technically legumes—and stay away from cashews because they contain more carbohydrates than any other nut.

NEVER CONSUME VEGETABLE OILS

Avoid vegetable oils entirely in your shopping and personal cooking, as these will inevitably be in your food whenever you eat out at restaurants. Never buy processed foods, which are loaded with vegetable oils.

AVOID LEGUMES

Legumes have carbohydrates, so it's best to avoid them. It also just so happens that a great deal of the population is allergic to legumes. So, it's best to also avoid eating beans, which isn't that hard. After all, I've never heard anyone say, "I'm really craving some beans!"

REPLACE TRADITIONAL FLOUR WITH ALMOND OR COCONUT FLOUR, BUT ONLY USE OCCASIONALLY

Remember, becoming unstoppable is a lifestyle—not a rigid code. What's nice about it is that if you occasionally wander outside the boundaries you've constructed for yourself, it's going to be okay. You'll still perform optimally if you're keeping yourself in check more often than not. For example, I want to still be able to occasionally consume foods that have an emotional connection to my childhood—things like cookies or cake or muffins—for celebrations or special occasions. When you want to consume sweets like these, try to utilize almond or coconut flour as a substitute during baking. You can even occasionally make pancakes that have a lower glycemic index using these ingredients. Stay away from cassava flour and other high-carb flours. This shouldn't be too much of an issue, though, since even when using the right flours, pancakes and similar foods shouldn't be a staple of your diet.

CONSUME PLENTY OF SALT

When you eat fewer carbs, you need more salt. Your body has to have salt for hydration because without the proper salt levels, it's difficult to consume the amounts of water you'll need on a diet like this. But it has to be natural—sea salt or pink Himalayan. Iodized table salt is highly refined and incredibly poor quality. It might sound crazy to read that consuming plenty of salt is good, since salt has been falsely linked to hypertension, but myths aside, you need salt in your diet. While there is *some* evidence that white iodized table salt increases blood sugar slightly, that's because our bodies weren't meant to consume that kind of salt to begin with. Consume the kind of salt your ancestors ate and you're good to go. Salt is also a cheap, easy supplement you can take, too.

EAT IN-SEASON, ORGANIC FOODS

I'm not as concerned about buying an organic product if something is encased in hard-skin or in a shell. For example, I find no reason to buy an organic avocado—with a ridiculously hard shell, it's unlikely that pesticides and other nonorganic matter will find their way inside of it. But if there's a food that doesn't have thick skin for natural protection, I try to find the organic item in the supermarket—*especially* if it's likely that the nonorganic item has been given pesticides or antibiotics. Nonetheless, you're not going to die or harm your health from eating healthy things like vegetables that are nonorganic.

AVOID GMO FOODS

One of the debates unfolding in nutrition is whether or not GMO (genetically modified) foods should be consumed. Though it's not realistic to make everything in your diet organic, try to avoid GMO foods whenever you can, especially when it comes to fruits and meats. Stand on the side of caution. Interestingly, the US is one of the few developed countries that still allows the sale of GMO fruits. Most developed countries have banned GMO foods for good. This fascinates me, and also raises a ton of questions about how the US thinks about our food supply. I prefer food in its most natural state. It's probably bad to start messing with the genetics of foods.

BE ON THE LOOKOUT FOR PASTURED FOODS

What is a "pastured food"? Good question. The simple answer is that a pastured food item has been allowed access to open pasture during at least some of its lifetime, if not all of it. Poultry that's "pastured" has spent time outside of a cage and has been encouraged to roam while still having shelter from inclement weather. Pastured is different from cage-free, by the way. Pasture-raised chickens, for example, means that the chickens are actually outside, roaming, and eating stuff off the ground—vegetables, fruit, worms, whatever it is they find. They're sometimes fed grains as well, but they're living as they would normally if they weren't producing eggs and meat for us to consume.

Cage-free simply means that the chickens didn't live in a cage.

As for beef, I prefer grass-fed beef over non-grass-fed, but I do have non-grass-fed beef products at my house. Like pastured poultry and pork, grass-fed beef is more expensive. But it's also closer to the meat that was consumed by our ancestors, since the animals they ate weren't living in captivity. Also, it's clearly not natural to feed cows grains to the point that they would die if not killed for meat first. Not to mention feedlot operations are bad for the environment, which is different than sustainably and ethically raised grass-fed beef. Pay attention to these things—they do matter.

NEVER BUY FARM-RAISED FISH

Most of the salmon that's consumed these days is farm-raised. And that's awful. Here's why: farm-raised salmon are stuck in underwater pens and force-fed food that they'd never eat in the wild[45]—things like grains and livestock products. In other words, fish are fed food that comes from dry land, *not* the ocean. This leads to a host of problems, but one of the most noticeable is that when they're killed, they aren't even the same color as other fish due to their diet. As a result, they're injected with dye to look more "natural." So, stick to purchasing wild-caught salmon. In general, stick to fish that are small and not high up on the food chain. I do eat tuna sometimes, which would be considered a big fish. But just know that because of its size, fish high up on the food chain consume lots of crap in their lifetime. Wild-caught salmon is probably the best type of fish for your nutrition because it is high in omega-3s, too.

STAY AWAY FROM CHEAP GRAINS LIKE WHEAT, CORN, AND SOY

This includes any organism that consumed wheat, corn, or soy in its lifetime. Why? The simple reality is that the food that animals eat in its lifetime is also what *you're* eating. That means that if a cow ate a bunch of grains that were filled with antibiotics, you're eating those antibiotics, too. The quality of the meat you consume is directly related to the quality of nutrition that the animal had, and

---

45   Juliette Steen, "Everything You Should Know About Salmon Farming," *Huffington Post*, November 11, 2016, https://www.huffingtonpost.com.au/2016/11/10/ everything-you-should-know-about-salmon-farming_a_21603450/.

the natural—or *unnatural*—conditions it lived in. Keep it local. Stay away from industrially raised meats. Carefully read the packaging on your meats, and, if possible, purchase meat from the counter that isn't packaged.

INTERMITTENTLY FAST

Humans evolved to fast. They did so out of necessity, sometimes going long periods of time before they were able to hunt and gather food. After all, our ancestors didn't have access to food the way we do nowadays. So it's beneficial to fast intermittently. In fact, there's science and data showing the benefits of fasting.[46] It lowers blood sugar, decreases insulin levels, reduces inflammation, and allows the body to reset insulin sensitivity for improved brain function. And the wonderful thing about fasting is that the results can be seen in a short amount of time. This means you can measure its impact on your optimization efforts almost right away. Fasting is also free and saves you money, since eating less food obviously costs less money. The easiest way to intermittently fast is to simply skip breakfast. Since these guidelines are part of a lifestyle, there's no need to fast during popular meals that might affect your social life.

---

46 Monique Tello, "Intermittent Fasting: Surprising Update," *Harvard Health Blog*, June 29, 2018, https://www.health.harvard.edu/blog/intermittent-fasting-surprising-update-2018062914156.

Curious about fasting? There's an entire bonus chapter on the topic over at www.unstoppablebook.com/bonus.

FINISH EATING AT LEAST THREE HOURS BEFORE BED

The best way to prepare your body for sleep is to stop eating three hours before bed. That's because sleep is restorative for your body, and during that time, it's doing quite a bit of repair, processing, and absorbing of nutrients. By eating close to your bedtime, you add yet another process—digestion—to the roster for no reason. What's more, eating close to your bedtime means you'll more than likely go to bed feeling full, and that has the potential to disrupt your sleep. By being intentional about what you eat and *when* you eat it, you'll stay in charge of your day.

CYCLE CARBS INTO YOUR DIET ON A MONTHLY OR QUARTERLY BASIS

To put it bluntly, occasionally cycling carbs into your diet lets your body know that it's not dying. If you're eating the same things all of the time and are in ketosis all the time, your body will get worried—it'll crave variation. For example, sometimes fruit or white rice cooked in coconut oil, butter, or MCT. The fat I cook the rice in slows digestion so that the carbs in the rice don't spike my blood sugar and minimizes the negative impact it has on my body. This is a safe way to cycle carbs into your diet. One caveat: I don't use cycling varieties of foods in and out of my diet as an excuse to eat whatever I want. You won't find me eating a big slice of pizza, for example, because gluten isn't part of the Unstoppable Lifestyle. Cycling isn't an excuse to eat junk.

MEAL PREP AND COOKING METHODS

Don't cook with oils that have low burn or smoke points. A good example of an oil that has a low burn or smoke point is olive oil. Everyone has been told that olive oil is healthy and that butter should be substituted with olive oil. But the truth is that when olive oil is cooked on medium to high heat, its components break down, and the oil becomes extremely unhealthy fat. In cooking with olive oil, we as a culture have taken something that's actually healthy for us and have destroyed it with heat.

Olive oil should only be used on cold foods, like salads or vegetables, or foods that are already prepared. If you're eating a piece of fish, for example, you can put olive oil on your plate for the fish because you aren't cooking with it. Instead, cook with butter, ghee, lard, tallow, or suet. If you don't like cooking with any of the items I just mentioned and you're looking for an olive oil substitute, your best bet is going to be avocado oil. This has become very popular and is available even in Costco. It has a high smoke and burn point and is safe to cook with.

Cook foods on low temperatures. Believe me, I like charred, blackened, and smoked foods as much as anyone. I recently moved to Austin, Texas, a hotbed for barbecue, which I've taken full advantage of in the past. But food that has been blackened, like smoked meats, is caused by oxidation, which creates inflammation in the body. This should be avoided. And so should beef jerky—a food that I've seen many people start eating because they think it's a "good source of protein." But this isn't accurate. Meat that has been smoked like this, one, creates an oxidative and inflammatory environment, and, two, cooks so long that it has no fat. Thus, your meat becomes a low-fat item. To add insult to injury, foods like this often contain hidden sugars or even refined sugars. Read the label carefully and go with a premium brand of jerky. Good jerky is a nice treat that I occasionally enjoy.

Steam vegetables and other foods instead of microwaving them or boiling them. Steaming vegetables helps them to maintain their nutrients. When reheating foods in general, I prefer to use a steam oven over a microwave. Microwaving might cause damage to the makeup of the food, but don't worry, it's not going to give you cancer.

The steam oven I have is, without a doubt, one of my top-five purchases and was not even that expensive compared with other things you might decide that you need on this journey. Plus, even though steaming takes longer and doesn't provide the same instant gratification of a microwave, it makes the food healthier and helps it taste better. Use the extra time that it takes to prep the right foods for other healthy activities like taking a few minutes to focus on your breathing and slowing things down. By slowing down or delaying the instant gratification we have come to expect with food, we take back control of our health. Try it.

FIND AND REMOVE FOODS THAT CAUSE ALLERGIC REACTIONS

Food allergies and sensitivities are annoying. They also cause inflammation in the body, which makes allergies more than just a nuisance—it makes them dangerous. Gluten is a good example of this. Though not everyone will experience a major allergic reaction to gluten consumption, the majority of people's bodies cannot handle it optimally. If you've even an inkling of a food allergy or sensitivity, I recommend you get tested for it. Even though they're only reliable 60 percent of the time, they'll catch major problems like gluten and dairy. There are also so-called "elimination diets" which allow you to isolate foods in order to figure out which ones could be causing problems. By identifying sensitivities like these, you'll be able to reduce or eliminate inflammation in your body so it doesn't have to work as hard to feel good. One quick caveat, though: don't just stop eating something because it says that you're sensitive. But if your results say that you're sensitive to eggs *and* you've been eating eggs your whole life, experiment with this notion. Maybe go a week without eating eggs and see how you feel. See if the quantitative and qualitative data align in your experimentation.

IS SNACKING OKAY WITHIN THE UNSTOPPABLE LIFESTYLE?

Back in the day, I was the king of snacking. I snacked all day and every day at Grasshopper. That's because I had read somewhere that snacking was healthy, and it was the only excuse I needed to vanquish the hunger I constantly felt. The great thing about the Unstoppable Lifestyle is that it fills this void as well: you naturally won't snack as much because you'll feel full more often.

So, can you still snack? The answer is yes. But implement mindful eating into your snacking habits. Are you eating just to eat, perhaps out of boredom or stress? Are you snacking even if you already feel full? Be aware of your body, mind, and emotions before deciding to snack. You might discover that your desire to eat is really just another emotion competing for your attention, and not driven by actual hunger.

Whenever I do snack these days, it's usually when I'm traveling. But I prepare for this ahead of time by throwing a couple even-boiled eggs (where you aren't killing all the nutrients in the yoke), some cheese, or an avocado in a small cooler. If that's too much for you, keep a small bag of nuts (like macadamia, pistachios, or almonds, whether dry-roasted, salted, or unsalted) in your bag. Just be careful with nut butters, however. A lot of nut butters on the market today have either sugar or oils in them to stabilize them. You want nut butters that are as pure as possible, and *not* 100 percent almond, since almonds are high in protein. I try to keep my snacks as close to the whole food and original state as possible. Jerky and snack bars are obviously foods that are very far from their original states. But I understand their appeal because they are packaged and easy to eat on the go. There *is* high-quality jerky out there that you can purchase (not the processed jerky that fills aisles in grocery and convenience stores) and snack bars that you can find as well—just do your homework to find the right ones. I recommend looking for healthier packaged snacks at Whole Foods or Trader Joe's—these ones say they're keto- or paleo-safe and call out that no sugar is added. But proceed with caution: look for fake sweeteners and certain flours that are sometimes used in production. Most importantly, be aware of the net carbs in these snacks, which you can find on their label. I've noticed that there are a couple of brands of snack bars I've had that, even though they are labeled "safe" ended up throwing me out of ketosis, so I stopped eating those.

Whenever I'm at home or in the office and want to snack, I'll sometimes make my own "fat bombs," which are made with things like coconut, ghee, butter, and other healthy fats, rolled up into a ball and perhaps combined with other tasty things like cacao. There are a number of different options for these fat bombs that you'll find with a quick internet search. There are even some that have 100 percent dark chocolate in them, which gives you the feeling that you're eating something like candy, although much healthier. Sometimes I'll even have a couple of spoonfuls of olive oil or avocado oil—and I've seen others eat butter straight (not for the faint of heart). This might not sound filling at all, but remember, your body is going to naturally turn these healthy fats into energy.

Chocolate is a good snack, too, but only *very* specific chocolates that have a high percentage of cacao. For some people, this kind of chocolate is difficult to eat, so there are some other brands that include some of the fake sugars and sweeteners in their cacao chocolate. Other brands combine this chocolate with coconut, coconut fat, or other paleo- and keto-safe ingredients that make them easier and tastier to consume. Cheese is also a reasonable, affordable snack. I prefer to stay away from dairy because my body, like most people's bodies, doesn't handle lactose well, but solid cheese that's unprocessed and is as close as possible to its original manufactured state can be a great, filling snack.

I've found that snacking is very personal and needs to be tested. I can give you snacking suggestions, but it would be ridiculous for me to tell you how much or how little you can snack, as a number of fad diets do. Fad diets can be attractive to some people because of their black-or-white, systematic approach to food, but the Unstoppable Lifestyle takes things much deeper and hinges upon your own experimentation. The reason for this is because black-and-white diets work for a little while, and might cause you to lose some weight, but they never make a difference in the long run. Like everything else within the framework, experiment with what works best for your body. Just be aware of your current physical, mental, and emotional state. All of these affect your eating and snacking habits.

IS THIS KIND OF LIFESTYLE EXPENSIVE?

By now you might be thinking to yourself, "Eating this way is going to cost too much." And while I can't deny it's going to be more expensive on a daily basis, it's going to save you money in the long run when you're able to avoid expensive prescriptions, trips to the doctor, and wasting money on the steady stream of "new" fad diets. By following the guidelines within the Unstoppable Lifestyle, the goal is to find the healthy eating habits that'll be easiest for you to maintain over the long term.

Also, know that if you follow these guidelines, you'll probably also be eating *less* food than before because you're consuming higher-quality items that are high in fat and can be more easily converted into energy. To put it simply, you'll get full, even while eating less food.

CAN YOU EAT OUT OR CELEBRATE SPECIAL OCCASIONS?

Unlike a lot of fad diets out there that are unnecessarily restrictive and, quite frankly, make you seem self-righteous, my message is to *enjoy life*. Don't be dogmatic. Don't be unreasonable. Just enjoy each day, make common-sense decisions, and don't be the jerk in the room that needs to have a special meal or a special dish. I encourage you *not* to take these Unstoppable Lifestyle guidelines from the last two chapters, or yourself, too seriously. You can't let them rule your life. Dedicate yourself to them, but don't burden your friends or family with your dietary needs. Don't bug others by demanding you eat special foods. If there's something on your plate that you know is going to drastically upset your body, just pick around it. Enjoy life, go out to dinner, attend family events, and have a glass of wine at a friend's house if you want. Trust me, your body will bounce back, especially if you're sticking to these guidelines for the majority of the time.

Enjoy special occasions. After all, they're "special" because they don't come around very often. If everyone is around for Christmas or Thanksgiving, eat the meal that's there and enjoy it. There's no need to feel guilty or ashamed about it. Now, if you're a person who's going over to people's houses for dinner parties two or three times a week, you might have to be more guarded to stay within the boundaries of your diet, but for me, I know that one day, or a couple of meals every month or two, isn't going to kill me.

That being said, I completely understand the anxiety that can sometimes, at first, come along with following guidelines like this, especially when it comes to things like traveling or eating out. Once again, just plan ahead. Take a small cooler. Bring a bag of nuts. If you're flying, go to a Whole Foods or grocery store right when you arrive at your destination—that's what I always do. Make this a part of your routine. At the store, stock up on things like avocados, eggs, cheese, and smoked salmon (none of which requires a lot of cooking) for your hotel refrigerator. Whole Foods will even cook the salmon for you. If you know you're going to be eating out, just remember that most restaurants are cooking with hidden sugars and vegetable oils and using cheap ingredients to compensate for their level of production. Even things like dressings and sauces, especially sauces that are spicy, will have sugars in them to create that feeling in your taste buds that gets you addicted and keeps you coming back. Just keep all of that in the back of your mind before you place your order. One of the reasons I don't eat vegetable oils at home is because I know I'm going to get them at restaurants. And I won't feel guilty for eating them at restaurants because I know I'm in control. Stay on top of your diet whenever you can, and it's going to allow you to be more flexible when you're eating out. This goes back to planning ahead.

Case in point: on a recent work trip to Boston, I knew we were going to go out to eat at least one night. Unsure what I'd be able to eat at the restaurant, I ate a couple of snacks from my refrigerator before going out, and then just ordered an appetizer at the restaurant. Rather than feeling frustrated at the lack of options specifically designed for me, I've learned to take control of my own fuel intake. And remember, control doesn't mean *restriction*. Control is the freedom from frustration. That evening, instead of being hungry and having to spend a ton of time sifting through the menu and asking the waiter all kinds of questions, I was able to be present with people and focus on the conversation that was unfolding, which is what's most important anyway. Plus, I wasn't the weirdo sitting at a table without food in front of me or having to answer questions from curious people about my diet.

Similarly, one of the things my family loves to do is go out for sushi. We go to the same place frequently—sometimes once a week—for our night out. Never in my wildest dreams could I imagine taking this tradition away from my family because of *my* diet or lifestyle. It's a shame that so many fad diets not only lead to frustration for the person adopting the diet (because of guilt and shame) but also for the people around them whom they love. If you're following a restrictive diet that makes you or others miserable, you're chasing the wrong outcome. Whenever we go out for sushi, I eat a regular meal, with rice, every single time. I enjoy it and I don't feel guilty at all. I'm in control of the decision, and I know that my body can handle it. I can make these decisions, enjoy life, and continue my journey.

Having control over my own fuel has produced an ever-expansive mental and emotional freedom within me. I'm more present with others. I can find the beauty in the present moment. That's what naturally happens when you're no longer wasting energy judging yourself. That's what happens when you've nothing but goodwill toward yourself. Things start to open up within you. You no longer live in fear or judgment or shame. You start enjoying your life and the many moments that are gifted to you every day.

These days I'm in full control of my fuel intake because of the mechanisms I've built into my routine, which has led to a freedom from frustration. Those clouds that once defined my journey are long gone. I haven't seen them in years. Frankly, I don't even know what guilt and shame feel like anymore because they're so foreign to my daily experience. You can see a lot more clearly when those clouds of guilt and shame are no longer looming over you.

KEY TAKEAWAYS

I can't emphasize enough how powerful the process of experimentation has been for me, and can be for you, too. Try these guidelines above and see how you feel. If you've already found a diet that works for you—whether it's keto, paleo, LCHF (low-carb high-fat), or even a vegan, plant-based diet—most of these guidelines can be used in tandem with that diet. Remember, this book isn't about following a strict set of rules; it's about finding what works for *you*. Fad diets will come and go, but discovering a health optimization strategy will serve you for the rest of your life.

The more you experiment, observe, and listen, the more you'll find that your body sends a lot of signals that can be used as inspiration for experiments. As you test new hypotheses, be aware and curious—try to pinpoint what improved within your body and connect it to the experiments you're running at that time. Remember, this isn't just about getting healthy; it's about becoming unstoppable. And that means continuous experimenting and learning.

Get more resources and information about the Unstoppable Lifestyle at www.unstoppablebook.com/chapter11.

CHAPTER 12

SUPPLEMENTATION AND VITAMINS

By now you can see that the Unstoppable Lifestyle isn't restrictive. It's not a set of strict rules. After all, that's debilitating. The last thing people need is yet another reason to judge themselves or feel guilt and shame. Every aspect of this lifestyle is designed to free you physically, mentally, and emotionally.

Since the framework isn't a strict set of rules to follow or foods to eat, everyone has different results. But the theme uniting everyone's efforts is the concept of forward progress, of optimizing your unique body to become unstoppable. Although I encourage you to experiment with all facets of your life, from fuel to exercise and beyond, I realize everyone must move at their own pace.

As you think through your optimization efforts, I urge you to consider experimenting with another area related to fuel and nutrition: vitamins and supplementation.

Throughout my own personal journey, the more I optimized my fuel intake, the more obsessed I became with finding other ways of propelling myself forward. When I discovered vitamins and supplements, I was excited to experiment with something that our ancestors never had access to, that could potentially take my health and well-being to the next level. But, like many people, I was genuinely confused about which vitamins and supplements I should take, and why. Were some brands better than others? Were there supplements I couldn't find in the drugstore that I should be taking? And, perhaps most importantly, what data were there—if any at all—to back up the claims some of these vitamin manufacturers make? Rather than tell you to try a bunch of things without giving you a reason why, I urge you to consider doing the following before taking any vitamins or supplements:

1. BEFORE YOU DO ANYTHING, GET A BASELINE BLOOD PANEL.

Baseline testing entails testing for more than just what's involved in a routine annual blood test, and is important to complete before you experiment with supplementation. That's because a baseline panel is going to serve as your starting point, or the "before" to your "after." If you don't have a baseline blood panel completed, it's going to be impossible to prove whether or not your experiments with vitamins and supplements had any impact on you physically. And really, what's the point of that? There are some areas within dieting and nutrition I've discussed where experimentation hinges upon how you feel, but smart supplementation relies on hard data for the most part and, to a lesser degree, nuanced anecdotal observation. As an example, if you're experimenting with a B12 supplement and have never done testing, you might be able to make vague conclusions like "I feel better" or "I have more energy," but if you get a blood test first, you might be able to actually confirm that you need to supplement with B12 because of the significant lack in vitamin B in your blood. What's more, establishing baselines allows you to track changes over time. For example, if through frequent supplementation your vitamin B levels rise to a level that's too high, you can supplement less frequently so that your numbers return to a healthy range. If you decided not to establish a baseline with a blood test at the outset of experimenting with supplements, you'd never be able to make these micro-optimizations. Once you take your blood test, there's something important to know about what your "numbers" mean. With this kind of blood test, you'll be measured on a scale—for example, average, above average, or below average. These levels are determined based on comparisons with other people's numbers from the same lab. It's like a weighted grade on a test that you took in school: if everyone performed poorly on the test, your "good" grade doesn't necessarily indicate that you mastered the content. This is important to understand about your blood test because you might have "average" numbers, indicating that you're okay, but those average numbers could simply be average in the context of an unhealthy population.

But here's the thing: if you've made it this far in the book, it's obvious that you aren't aiming for normal or average. You're aiming for *optimal*. Blood tests can be expensive if you go beyond what your insurance allows (which isn't much, and frankly, is not all that helpful other than telling you whether or not you're dying). I also know that blood tests can cause anxiety for some people. But stay the course if supplementation interests you. If it doesn't interest you, you aren't going to die if you don't supplement. Thoughtful supplementation rooted in your baseline blood tests (like your vitamin panel) should only have positive effects with very little or no downsides. Because of this notion, know that you can easily read this chapter without taking action immediately. Consume the information, see if you get curious about it, and file it away with your growing list of things to test.

2. PAY ATTENTION TO QUALITY AND PURITY.

Once you get your baseline blood tests and develop a hypothesis to test within the framework that is rooted in the data you gathered, you can begin experimentation. You'll find at the start that the world of supplementation—which is already tremendously confusing and difficult—becomes even more cluttered when you start evaluating the different brands within each supplement. Look for brands that have the most "base" ingredients— no additional items. There are a number of brands that promote their base ingredients, but more importantly, find one that works for you and your body. Once your experimentation is based on hard data, you can start becoming more subjective about how different brands make you feel. Honestly, most of the core ingredients in supplements are purchased from a few main worldwide suppliers. Everything else comes down to:

- Pricing and packaging
- Quality
- Whether or not the company is buying from the original producer or another distributor

Any additives or cutting agents are usually represented in the price. I wouldn't necessarily recommend buying the most expensive brand, but I definitely wouldn't buy the cheapest brand. In this sense, I view supplements the way I view food—the cheaper the supplement, the further it is from its base ingredients.

3. TARGET YOUR SOLUTIONS.

Make sure that you stick to supplements that are for *one* vitamin. Experimentation can be difficult when you start playing around with "stacks," which are combined supplements, like multivitamins. It makes it difficult to identify your solutions. Here's why:

- The ingredients' bioavailability decreases when supplements are combined.
- They're usually more expensive: you can, for example, purchase D3 combined with K2, but it's actually cheaper to buy them separately.
- Most importantly, it's difficult to get your numbers to optimal levels when you're taking these combinations. For example, you might need to cut back on D3 intake yet maintain the steadiness of K2, but because they're combined, it's impossible to do so.

The truth is, you lose all control of influencing your numbers when supplements are combined. What's more, if you're being meticulous in your experimentation—like I am—taking a combined multivitamin is troublesome because you're relying on the manufacturer's ability to include the right amount of each individual vitamin in a multi, and sometimes that's *way* off. For those reasons, it's best to stick with base ingredients.

CRUCIAL SUPPLEMENTS

Supplementation can be an incredibly helpful part of building your Unstoppable Lifestyle. That's because our modern lives have left us nutritionally deficient in a number of ways. In order to recover from what's lacking in our diet, it's essential that you consider integrating the following vitamins and supplements into your routine.

D3

Vitamin D is a hormone responsible for metabolizing calcium, as well as absorbing iron, magnesium, phosphorous, and zinc.[47] Technically, it's a family of compounds, but the most important one is D3. We can generate vitamin D when our bodies are exposed to sunlight and when we eat the right foods. Some studies have also shown that vitamin D even helps to increase testosterone.[48] Over the years, the role of vitamin D in boosting the immune

---

47   Leigh Cowart, "The Weird History of Vitamin D—And What It Actually Has to Do with Sun," *Washington Post*, May 12, 2016, https://www.washingtonpost.com/news/speaking-of-science/wp/2016/05/12/the-weird-history-of-vitamin-d-and-what-it-actually-has-to-do-with-sun/?noredirect=on&utm_term=.a2ba0a5ca39d.

48   "Can Vitamin D Increase Testosterone Concentrations in Men?" *CATIE Treatment Update* 185 (2011), https://www.catie.ca/en/treatmentupdate/treatmentupdate-185/nutrition/can-vitamin-increase-testosterone-concentrations-men.

system and fighting heart disease and cancer[49] has been well documented, too. Problem is, vitamin D is also *really* hard to get from diet alone. Fatty fish are a good source—think salmon and tuna—but other than that, if you want vitamin D, you're going to need to take a supplement.

Back in the day, our ancestors didn't have supplements, so they got vitamin D naturally—from sunlight and consuming the fatty foods that were readily available to them. But today, we don't spend nearly as much time in the sunlight, and due to decades of misinformation, we avoid fatty foods that naturally contain the vitamin D our bodies require. The convergence of these events has created a vitamin D deficiency that impacts 41.6 percent of the US general population.[50]

When vitamin D has so much potential to benefit the population, it's unfortunate so few people are aware of the power of this supplement. But here's the good news: you can take the steps needed to incorporate vitamin D into your routine for very little investment up front. Just purchase 360 high-potency pills—they'll last you the entire year, and they'll cost you less than buying sixty high-quality omega-3 fish oil pills. Of course, I still urge

---

49 "Vitamin D and Health," Harvard School of Public Health, https://www.hsph.harvard.edu/nutritionsource/vitamins/vitamin-d/.

50 K. Y. Forrest and W. L. Stuhldreher, "Prevalence and Correlates of Vitamin D Deficiency in US Adults," *Nutrition Research* 31, no. 1 (2011): 48–54, doi: 10.1016/j.nutres.2010.12.001

you to take the extra time to research any supplement brand you're interested in taking to identify the quality of the base ingredients. Avoid buying the cheapest option—most vitamin D is already pretty inexpensive, so it's worth paying a few extra bucks for something good.

And, like everything else, I recommend testing for D3. A simple 25-hydroxy vitamin D (calcifediol) blood test will help you determine how much vitamin D is in your body (optimal levels of D3 in the blood are around 60 to 80 ng/mL and maybe more, depending on the guidelines you follow). If your D3 levels are low, which is likely, I recommend doubling or tripling your D3 intake from the start, just for the sake of experimentation. Then, get another blood test to check your numbers. If you need to, increase the dosage. This is a decent strategy if you really want to find a dosage that works for you. But remember, you need a baseline *and* consistent testing to accurately track changes.

B12

Just like D3, most people are also pretty low in B12, the vitamin that's found in animal products—including fish, meat, poultry, eggs, and milk products. Deficiencies in B12 can result in low energy, brain fog, and stiffness or weakness in limbs or muscles. B12 is a base vitamin that's essential for your body. Most people are pretty low in B12, even those who regularly consume animal products. B12 isn't fat soluble like D3, meaning that it's not absorbed better when consumed with fat. Your body will naturally excrete whatever you don't need.

One of the differences is the B12 supplements may be taken sublingually, meaning that it's a pill that melts in your mouth, rather than being swallowed. Many people prefer this method because it potentially allows for faster absorption and increased uptake. Although there's no proof that this is better, I've certainly found that sublingual B12 is a lot easier to take on the go. In addition to B12, you can also take a B-complex capsule that adds balance to the full spectrum of vitamin B in your body. One last note: a lot of times you'll find B12 combined with methylfolate, which, again, I wouldn't recommend taking, since it's difficult to isolate the impact of the combined supplement. That is, if you begin to take one and see a change in your blood tests, it's hard to say which part of the combined supplement made an impact. B12 is a little bit more expensive than D3, but it's still not a high-end supplement. The impacts of B12 supplementation are, however, on the same level as D3, making it well worth your time, money, and energy.

OMEGA-3 FISH OIL

You've probably heard a lot about this supplement. After

multivitamins, omega-3 fish oil is one of the supplements getting the most buzz today. But because of this, a lot of people are making mistakes with it. Before we dig in on what exactly people are doing wrong with omegas, let me explain what they are and how they work.

Omega-3s are fatty acids that are used for energy, tissue, and cell maintenance throughout your body. There are three types: alpha-linolenic acid (ALA), eicosapentaenoic acid (EPA), and docosahexaenoic acid (DHA). According to the National Institutes of Health, "DHA levels are especially high in retina (eye), brain, and sperm cells. Omega-3s also provide calories to give your body energy and have many functions in your heart, blood vessels, lungs, immune system, and endocrine system (the network of hormone-producing glands)."[51]

Even though omega-3s are incredibly powerful, most people don't get enough of them in their diet. That's because omega-6s dominate the average American diet in the form of cheap oils that are added to just about everything. When consumed unchecked, omega-6s can undercut the performance of any omega-3s we consume. For this reason, it's critically important to balance the amount of both omega-3s and omega-6s in our diet.

---

51 "Omega-3 Fatty Acids," National Institutes of Health, November 21, 2018, https://ods.od.nih.gov/factsheets/Omega3FattyAcids-Consumer/.

Even if you consume a lot of salmon or fish, chances are high you're *still* not consuming enough omega-3s. That's because most of the omega oils people consume are actually omega-6, coming from vegetable oils and other ingredients like that. In general, most people need to decrease their omega-6 consumption and increase their omega-3 consumption, though healthy levels of both do point toward benefits in heart health in the long-term. Compared with other supplements like D3 and B12, omegas are different because of their potential for these long-term benefits and effects. In the short term, many people have also noticed a difference in their skin, hair, and nails while taking omega-3 fish oil.

I've included omega-3 in the first tier of supplementation recommendations because, like the others I've mentioned, it's lacking in the majority of people's diets. It's also afford-able, in part due to increased availability and competition on websites like Amazon. For this supplement, pay atten-tion to the quality of ingredients. A lot of supplement manufacturers are purchasing the base product from a facility, which isn't the same as coming straight from a wild animal. That's why I personally prefer krill oil, specifically Antarctic krill oil. This product includes the most complete set of fats because they use the *whole* fish, not just parts of it.

What's the deal with using parts of fish to produce omega-3 supplements?

Manufacturers of lower-quality or "supermarket" omega-3 supplements use this practice because it's *cheap*. You get less of the good stuff inside of the fish and they get more profit.

With this method of manufacturing omega-3, instead of using the entire fish, fat is extracted from the skin. Many of these extractions come from farm-raised fish, which, as I mentioned earlier, already face terrible conditions in captivity. Remember how their flesh is dyed pink at the end of being "raised" so that it looks like a normal piece of salmon? That's the quality of fish that the majority of omega-3 supplements are being harvested from. Doesn't sound too appealing, and it's definitely not healthy.

Even if it's more expensive, I like knowing that my Antarctic krill oil is coming from wild fish, not a farm-raised salmon or similar. Frankly, it's questionable whether or not farm-raised fish even *contain* beneficial omega-3s. You see, if a fish is being deprived of its natural habitat and diet—the very habitat and diet that has led to their being rich in essential fatty acids in the first place—it stands to reason that farm-raised fish lack exposure to the very elements that make them so healthy. Particularly if, as is the case with most farm-raised salmon, they're fed a terrestrial diet consisting of everything from poultry to grain.

Think about it: with this supplement, producers are

taking a fish and breaking it down to its fundamental components, the fatty oils within it. Any environmental or nutritional problems that the fish had in its lifetime will inevitably come out in the product and into your body.

I prefer to get a complete set of high-quality fats when I take an omega-3 supplement, and I certainly don't want the fatty acids I'm consuming to come from a fish raised in captivity and fed food that's grown on *land*. Cheap omega-3s don't help you in the long run because the manufacturing process has been corrupted, and they're devoid of nutritional value. Avoid them.

A quick word about testing and evaluating the impact of high-quality omega-3 supplements. In general, it's hard to track the effects of this supplement in the blood. If you want to measure its efficacy, I recommend you leverage omega-3 to omega-6 ratios and fat in the stool.

PREBIOTICS AND PROBIOTICS

Your gut is incredibly important to the health of your body and mind. When the organisms inside of your gut are thrown out of balance by external forces, it can wreak havoc on your digestion and even your mood.[52] That's

---

52 "Prebiotics, Probiotics and Your Health," Mayo Clinic, March 6, 2018, https://www.mayoclinic. org/prebiotics-probiotics-and-your-health/art-20390058.

why it's important to understand the role of two key drivers of gut health: prebiotics and probiotics.

Prebiotics, which are found in things like chicory and fermented foods, are specialized plant fibers that help to grow healthy bacteria in the gut. Probiotics are live bacteria and yeasts that are good for your digestion. Some are formulated into capsules or added to certain foods and beverages. Just like fuel, though, it's always best to get your prebiotics in their most natural or whole form, so I recommend you try to get prebiotics in the food you eat.

While gut health is important, it's also a burgeoning area of study. As a result, there are few conclusive studies on its efficacy. Research doesn't exactly say *why* probiotics are good other than the fact that the stomach and intestines need a variety of different flora, bacteria, and bio-essences for balance. But the benefits of probiotics are wide-ranging,[53] as they've been shown to alleviate symptoms of ulcerative colitis (UC), irritable bowel syndrome (IBS), Crohn's, urinary tract infections (UTI), and many other health problems.

Personally, probiotics have had a tremendously positive impact on my health. When purchasing, I look for two

---

[53] "Health Benefits of Taking Probiotics," Harvard Health Publishing, last modified August 22, 2018, https://www.health.harvard.edu/vitamins-and-supplements/health-benefits-of-taking-probiotics.

things: first, that they're refrigerated (which, by the way, makes this supplement challenging to travel with), and second, that the brand is used to help with UC, Crohn's, or IBS. There are only a few brands that have actually been scientifically proven to help with these diseases, and therefore those are the brands I tend to use.

Keep in mind: there are lots of options out there with probiotics and therefore lots of claims, but very few brands are scientifically backed, since this area is still relatively new. I usually take one probiotic a day. But frequency will hinge upon your own experimentation. Overall, this is something that has higher impact, but is also much higher cost—probably as expensive as the previous three supplements combined. If you decide to experiment with probiotics, it'll be up to you to gather more research, keep your eye out for new scientific studies, and decide what works for you.

IMPORTANT SUPPLEMENTS

Our bodies can be improved with the help of various supplements. Since I believe some supplements can be more beneficial than others, I've sorted them into the categories you see in the book: Crucial, Important, and Other Supplements to Consider. I urge you to experiment in the order that makes the most sense for you, and, of course, not all at once.

FIBER

Fiber cleanses and removes toxins from your body. It's mostly found in green, leafy vegetables, and that's my personal preference for getting sufficient fiber in my diet. As I mentioned, consuming whole foods is usually the best way to get the nutrients your body needs. However, it's worth considering supplementing with fiber because it's such an essential nutrient for your body to operate efficiently.

I get it, though—fiber scares people. There are so many horror stories about disruptive trips to the bathroom after taking so-called "fiber pills" and the like. But those situations are usually a by-product of industrial-strength fiber pills that function more like laxatives. Instead of products like that, I prefer a fiber supplement called psyllium husk, which doesn't contain any carbs. It's also way more gentle—nothing like what you might see on the grocery shelf, which is designed to clean you out quickly. Psyllium husk should hardly affect the frequency of your bowel movements but will also remove toxins from your body.

Fiber is also great when used in tandem with probiotics and prebiotics, as it's needed in your stomach and intestines for both of those to function properly. On top of that, fiber is dirt cheap. A huge bottle of psyllium husk is ten dollars, which is even less expensive than the highest-quality D3 supplements.

MAGNESIUM

Magnesium is a core component of several key processes within the human body. You might find that supplementing with magnesium will help you sleep more soundly and think more clearly. But because of its numerous functions within the body, magnesium comes in many different forms: you can take it in pill form, drink it by mixing powder into a beverage, add it to your food, or rub it on your skin. There are even sensory deprivation tanks where you essentially float in a salt-magnesium bath. While I can't tell you which form of magnesium will be best for you, I can say that it's worth your experimentation.

As you research and start to test different types of magnesium, ask yourself:

- **Which form of magnesium might be the best to start out with?**
- For some people, taking a pill is easier, while others don't mind mixing the powder into a drink.
- **Are you sleeping more or getting better sleep while testing a specific type of magnesium?**
- When experimenting with different types of magnesium, track the same things for consistency (quantity and quality of sleep, and so on).
- **How's your brain function?**
- Is it easier to concentrate? Can you concentrate for

longer? How's your memory? Track what you find
valuable.

- **What's your mood like?**
- Is there any relationship between taking magnesium,
  sleeping more soundly, and your behavior during the
  day?

Sometimes people experience muscle cramps or headaches when on magnesium supplements, so be aware
of those potential negative effects and take them into
account in your experimentation and data collection.

VITAMIN C

For decades, people have been told that vitamin C primarily comes through consuming fruits, but it's simply
not true. You can get vitamin C from a number of other
food products, including vegetables and meats. I avoid
vitamin C packets that you mix into a beverage because
the powder usually consists of other ingredients besides
vitamin C, sometimes sugar.

There are studies that show that vitamin C supplementation can help with the absorption of other types of
nutrients, but I personally don't find a need to supplement
with vitamin C. I know I'm getting enough through the
food I consume. Like magnesium, this is a supplement
that's based on how you feel subjectively. Personally, it

hasn't helped me to feel any better or worse. If you're taking many other supplements, however, it might be worth adding. It's cheap and has relatively few negative side effects.

SALT

In following the Unstoppable Lifestyle, a high-fat diet will likely result in your body lacking in salt. I thought I was putting enough salt into my food, but it's actually hard to do when following a high-fat diet. So, I began taking a salt hydration supplement. I stay away from salt supplements that have calcium citrate.

If you're following one of the diets I discussed and it's something you think you'll follow on a long-term basis, a salt supplement is probably something that you need to look into. It's cheap and easy to test with. Simply try it for a few days and see how you feel. If you don't feel significantly better, it's probably not worth your time and energy.

OTHER SUPPLEMENTS TO CONSIDER

There are so many supplements out there for you to experiment with, but this last group is comprised of more uncommon recommendations. And, unlike the two groups of supplements I shared earlier, this list contains some that might have undesirable side effects. This will require you to proceed with awareness and caution. What's more, before you can even consider the supplements in this list, please try the ones in the first two groups first. This will allow you to get accustomed to the process of experimenting with supplements and monitoring how your body reacts to them.

So, what's the potential upside?

Well, there's plenty. But you have to work up to this stage of experimentation and be open to a fair amount of sophisticated testing and analysis. That's because these supplements are also relatively emergent, and there's just not a lot of research out there to help narrow our focus.

In the next few sections, I'll give you a rough overview of what I view to be the primary three supplements in this category: nootropics, pharmaceuticals, and mind-altering or psychotropic substances. There are tons of other supplements that also fall into this category, but instead of listing all of those here, I've streamlined it down to the three that I think are most important:

- *Nootropics*: These are known as "smart drugs" or cognitive enhancers, and they're designed to enhance brain function—memory, focus, clarity, and the like.

There's a bit of evidence that these might be effective, but the data is still inconclusive. These drugs are highly combined, and since there's no research on long-term effects of nootropics, experiment with them *at your own risk*. Because of the varied ingredients in nootropics, you might find that your numbers might get thrown out of whack. If you're keeping strict data, as I do, you'll find that nootropics will make it difficult for you to manage your numbers. I personally stay away from nootropics, but this is certainly a category that's worth knowing about.

- *Pharmaceuticals:* This is an obvious one. As a society, we're generally very comfortable as a population taking—and trusting—pharmaceuticals. You might not consider this supplementation, but it is: you're taking a pill to supplement your body with something it's supposedly lacking. Though it happens to be pharmaceutical in origin, there are a number that are beneficial for people. For example, there are drugs that lower blood sugar along with others that have positive long-term effects. Pharmaceuticals are definitely on the more extreme side of supplementation because you often have to get a doctor involved, and there are potentially more negative side effects. I'd look into these if I couldn't solve my medical problems otherwise, but my preference is to do everything without the aid of pharmaceuticals. Remember, these drugs usually mask the symptoms rather than address the root cause of an issue. But as a last resort, pharmaceuticals can be useful.

- *Psychotropic substances*: These are chemical substances that change the way your brain functions. Sometimes they're recommended by a psychiatrist to treat mental illness. Other times they're used for recreational purposes. Psychotropics are an area in which there's still a lot of research to be done. It's worth keeping an eye on this research in the future, but, like nootropics, the lack of existing research into long-term effects is a red flag. At the very least, because of this, they shouldn't be used frequently or without the recommendation of a medical professional. I encourage you to research them more and contemplate how they might benefit you before experimenting.

KEY TAKEAWAYS

My health and wellness journey has given me the chance to explore a lot of potential areas of optimization related to vitamins and supplementation. From omega-3s and vitamin D to probiotics and psychotropics, there's a ton of things you can test, measure, and evaluate. Rather than go down that road alone, I've provided you with the key areas worth your time and attention, as well as areas that may require a more cautionary approach. While experimenting in this realm of the Unstoppable Lifestyle, I urge you to use a methodical approach and educate yourself, or consult the help of a professional before trying something new. The goal here is to become a better version of yourself—the unstoppable version—so that you can lead as full a life as possible.

If you're curious and want to learn more, it's helpful to learn how these vitamins and supplements have impacted others. There are Reddit subs and other types of discussion groups out there where people talk about what they've tried and the effects of certain supplements. While this isn't scientific, it could help to point you in the right direction for experimentation or further inquiry.

CHAPTER 13

SLEEP

When I was a kid, my mom used to tell me how important it was to get enough sleep. This sentiment was echoed regularly on the news and in other popular media. But, when I was young, the most important thing to me was work. I wanted to start a company—there was no time for sleep, I thought. Looking back, it's kind of amusing, but I also realize it's incredibly common. Many of us sacrifice healthy habits to pursue other goals, dreams, or outcomes. Maybe you can relate. Is there something else in your life that has always taken precedence over the core aspects of your own health?

When we started Grasshopper, my co-founder and I were in college full time. Despite this, we provided 24/7 customer service to small businesses, and incoming calls went directly to my cell phone. I would answer every call—

even if it was in the middle of the night! My phone was always next to my pillow. Whether or not the calls came in, I always had the expectation that it *could* happen, and as a result, I never felt like I got great sleep.

Grasshopper continued to grow rapidly in my early twenties. And, although customer service calls no longer went straight to my phone, I'd work each day until I physically couldn't anymore. Exhausted, I'd come home from the office, and, within minutes, fall asleep on my couch for about an hour. I'd then wake up and go upstairs to my office and work for another three or four hours. Sleep, as I've mentioned, was something I thought I could get caught up on when I was dead. I was determined to get things done, even if it meant sacrificing rest. To compensate, during the day, I ate whatever and whenever I felt like it. At night, I'd sleep only when I couldn't push my body any further. This, I thought, was what it took to be successful. It's no wonder I got several horrible colds each year. My immune system was incredibly weak because of how little recovery sleep I was getting.

Over time, a few bad habits had become a way of life for me. But I didn't seem to notice—after all, I thought I was doing what I had to do to be a successful entrepreneur. Plus, I was eating well (or so I thought) and working out more than ever. Looking back, I realize that so much of health is sticking to the basics: getting adequate sleep, treating your body gently, and eating whole foods. While I don't deny that starting a business requires long hours and a lot of work, and probably some sleepless nights, I can't help but wonder how much more optimal I could've been had I been focused on the basics and taking better care of myself. I wanted to be unstoppable, and thought I was—for a time. But because of my lack of sleep and poor diet, it eventually caught up with me. I regularly experienced frequent brain fog and, at times, struggled to focus. Nowadays, I understand how incredibly difficult it is to tap into the fullness of your mind and creativity when your body is always on the verge of shutting down due to exhaustion.

Just as I used to think that I needed to be constantly hungry in order to lose weight, I used to think that I needed to be constantly exhausted in order to be productive and be a good parent. In reality, the opposite was true: optimizing your work isn't about the number of hours you put in. It's about the *quality* of the hours you work. These days, I've a better work ethic than before because I'm maximizing more of my potential throughout the workday. I can be more present with the task at hand. I can be more focused. I can get lost in the workday and then shut things down when it's time to move on. Similar to working, being exhausted doesn't make you a good parent. Being *present* makes you a good parent. How are you supposed to be present if your body is out of whack or you're always desperate for energy?

As funny as it may sound, getting adequate sleep is essential if you want to become unstoppable. That's because sleep is restorative for both your body and mind. Getting good sleep helps you focus, make better decisions, and allows you to be more present in your relationships and daily activities. Today, I sleep twice as much as I used to, and my hours awake are five times more productive and beneficial.

But it wasn't always obvious to me how powerful sleep could be. If you're still in that frame of mind, the next few pages are designed for you. Getting adequate and consistent amounts of sleep, as you'll soon find out, is one of the most important steps we can take toward truly making ourselves unstoppable.

AN INTRODUCTION TO SLEEP

All animals sleep.

But humans are the *only* animals known to delay sleep in pursuit of other activities.

And we're pretty creative about it, too: we spend time endlessly scrolling through social media on our phones, browsing websites, watching movies, gaming, going out at night, working late, and so on. While a late night here and there certainly won't kill you, not getting adequate sleep on a regular basis has the potential to seriously undermine your health, and in a variety of ways. Besides zapping your energy during the day, chronic lack of sleep can impact mood and lead to memory problems, poor decision-making, hormonal disturbances, and headaches, as well as the development of inflammation in the body and an increased risk for metabolic syndrome disease in otherwise healthy individuals.[54] To put it simply, not getting enough sleep can have a very serious impact on your health.

Despite this, sleep is an area many people struggle to regulate. Some people even believe they've *adapted* to chronic lack of sleep and have resigned themselves to caffeinating and medicating their way around the grogginess and brain fog that accompanies it. In my early twenties when I was growing Grasshopper, that was definitely me. But as I've learned, life without the right amount of sleep won't allow you to live your life to the fullest—or healthiest.

So, how do you know if you're getting the right amount

54   Janet M. Mullington, Norah S. Simpson, Hans K. Meier-Ewert, and Monika Haack, "Sleep Loss and Inflammation," Best Practice & Research: Clinical Endocrinology & Metabolism 24, no. 5 (2010): 775-784, doi: 10.1016/j.beem.2010.08.014

of sleep? Easy. Just ask yourself the following question when you wake up: do I feel rested and ready for a new day? If your answer isn't "Hell yes!" then you've got some work to do.

It's okay, though—you're not alone. Research shows that around seventy million adults in the US suffer from sleep disorders.[55] Which isn't surprising, since we humans have practically made an art form of delaying natural sleep with all of the distractions we have around us. However, despite their allure, none of those distractions will be able to put back into your life all that they take away from it. That's why, if you really want to become unstoppable, you've got to make a commitment to optimizing your sleep.

In this chapter, I'll be exploring the different aspects of sleep optimization so that you can capitalize on one of the most vital sources of better health. What's more, sleep is one of the main areas where there's the potential for a huge return on your investment of time and effort. That's because chronic lack of sleep can impact everything from your ability to make better choices related to your diet and having enough energy to move your body, to reducing inflammation and decreasing your risk for metabolic

---

55   Emily Carlson, Alisa Machalek, Kirstie Saltsman, and Chelsea Toledo, "Tick Tock: New Clues about Biological Clocks and Health," National Institute of General Medical Sciences, November 1, 2012, https://www.nigms.nih.gov/education/Inside-Life-Science/Pages/Tick-Tock-New-Clues-About-Biological-Clocks-and-Health.aspx.

disorders. Nail this part of your health, and you'll find yourself functioning better in every other aspect of your life, too.

RHYTHMS, STAGES, AND CYCLES

The definition of "optimal sleep" is different for everyone, and that's why experimentation plays such a powerful role in determining the right amount of sleep for your body. In addition to optimizing your actual *quantity* of sleep, I urge you to consider optimizing your sleep *environment* as well. I've found that these two elements really go hand in hand because your environment plays a huge role in producing the conditions ideal for rest. Before we dig into recommended experiments in this area, though, it's helpful to understand three powerful components of sleep:

- Rhythms
- Stages
- Cycles

RHYTHMS

All humans follow a "circadian rhythm" that dictates when we go to sleep, when we wake up, and when we eat. Our circadian rhythm is dictated by tons of internal "biological clocks" made of proteins that interact with various cells[56] and live in every tissue and organ in our body. One giant "master clock" made up of 20,000 neurons[57] coordinates all these clocks, allowing masterful alignment of all of the different moving pieces. It's a beautiful thing.

While the circadian rhythm we follow is produced in large part by natural processes in the human body,[58] it can also be influenced by external forces, like light. For millions of years, our ancestors evolved in response to the largest natural source of external light there is, the sun. It dictated sleeping patterns by interacting with our optic nerve, which sends a signal to the brain to go to sleep.

But a funny thing has started to happen in recent history: in addition to responding to natural light sources like the sun, our bodies have begun responding to artificial sources of light like computer, phone, and television screens. By interacting with our optic nerves, these artificial sources of light are able to send signals to our brain to delay sleep.

You've probably experienced the effects of this exact scenario firsthand: you've had a long day at work, come

---

56   "Circadian Rhythms," National Institute of General Medical Sciences, last modified August 2017, https://www.nigms.nih.gov/education/pages/Factsheet_CircadianRhythms.aspx.

57   "Brain Basics: Understanding Sleep," National Institute of General Medical Sciences, last modified February 8, 2019, https://www.ninds.nih.gov/Disorders/Patient-Caregiver-Education/Understanding-Sleep.

58   "Circadian Rhythms."

home and have dinner, and decide to spend some time catching up on email. Half an hour later, you no longer feel as tired as you did when you came home. In fact, it feels like you're getting your second wind! So you spend some more time on email, watch some videos, and maybe browse a few websites, too. And, before you know it, it's incredibly late. Besides being terribly confusing for your body—which is trying very hard to prepare itself for rest—situations like this are actively withholding the release of melatonin, resetting our natural circadian rhythm, and changing our bodies. Over time, this can have massively negative effects on a host of physiological processes, including the regulation of hormones like cortisol, leptin, and ghrelin.

So, what should you do? Go to bed early and get up early.

Sounds extreme, but if you're trying to tap into your body's natural circadian rhythm, there's really no need to ever go to bed later than 9:00 or 9:30, the latest. In general, the more you can get back in line with the rising and setting of the sun, the more you'll tap into your body's natural routine. But no matter the schedule you establish, try to stick to it on weekends, too. The more your body becomes patterned, the more you'll optimize your quality of sleep. I know it's tempting to stick to this strategy only on weekdays and then nix it on the weekends, but it doesn't work (I've tried it). Keep things consistent seven days a week and your body will reward you.

The more you can stay on the same pattern and schedule, the more you'll wake up naturally, without the aid of an alarm clock. Aim for eight to nine hours per night. Personally, I go to bed at the same time every night, and there are very few circumstances where I've got to use an alarm because I get up so early every day. If, say, I have an early flight, I might set a backup alarm—just in case—but I honestly can't remember the last time that an alarm woke me up. My body is in its natural rhythm and, as a result, wakes up when it's *supposed* to wake up. If you're interested in experimenting with this (and I highly recommend you do), aim to implement this practice for a few weeks while tracking how your body feels at one-week intervals. What changes do you feel outside of simply getting more sleep? Are you more productive at work? Do you have a better ability to focus?

For more in-depth info on testing and tracking, head to www.unstoppablebook.com/bonus.

STAGES

There are three different stages of sleep: REM, deep sleep, and light sleep. When you sleep for a total of nine hours, you cycle through all three stages multiple times.

While it's well established that humans cycle through each stage while sleeping, what's not clear is how much sleep you need in each stage for optimal rest. Sleep aids and drugs affect these stages and so does your bedtime. That's because the most restorative and important sleep happens between 9:00 p.m. and 1:00 a.m.—and those are absolute times. You don't get the same benefits if you go to bed at 11:00 p.m. and sleep just as long—you miss out on the deep sleep. It's a phenomenon that goes back to how humans evolved.

There are some arguments about whether or not sleep stages are important, but I track them because I was one of those people who often woke up feeling like I wasn't well-rested or rejuvenated, even after eight or nine hours of sleep. I participated in both in-lab and at-home clinical testing, tracking sleep every night for more than a year. I continue to track sleep with my Oura ring because some of the deeper information has been interesting, but the most important measurement is simply how you feel in the morning. We'll talk more about tracking later, but generally speaking, the more REM and deep sleep you can get, the better. Here are some practical tips for optimizing your sleep rhythms and stages.

STAY AWAY FROM BLUE LIGHT BEFORE GOING TO BED

Blue light is mostly emitted by electronics. During the day, blue wavelengths keep us alert and help us pay attention,[59] but at night, they send signals to your brain to stay awake. Unsurprisingly, this makes it difficult for people to fall asleep.

If you've got to work late on your computer, there are tools you can install that'll block blue light from affecting your eyes so close to bedtime. And, yes, blue light also includes television. Because of this, I removed the television from my bedroom. Your television isn't going to help you get into deep cycles of sleep. If you do need to look at a screen before bed, perhaps for work or something else, either wear blue-light blocking glasses, or, much easier than that, install a program like f.lux or Iris on your computer. Both of these tools have a setting that adjusts the light given off depending on the time of day. For the phone, you can turn the brightness down and/or use a similar program to f.lux or Iris that adjusts the colors of your display to the warmer end of the color spectrum, making it easier on your eyes (on the iPhone, this is called Night Shift).

---

59 "Blue Light Has a Dark Side," Harvard Health Publishing, last modified August 13, 2018, https://www.health.harvard.edu/staying-healthy/blue-light-has-a-dark-side.

DON'T EAT WITHIN THREE HOURS OF BEDTIME

We eat to have fuel for activities that expend energy throughout the day. At night, as our bodies prepare for sleep, there's no reason to eat as if you're going to remain active. After all, you're about to lie down for eight or nine hours! Give your body a break by avoiding food within three hours of your bedtime. Your digestion will be better, and you'll sleep more soundly.

GO TO SLEEP BETWEEN NINE AND TEN O'CLOCK AT NIGHT, OR EARLIER

Our ancestors' deepest sleep occurred between 9:00 p.m. and 1:00 a.m., and to this day, we follow this pattern. That's why going to bed between nine and ten at night is ideal.

WAKE UP BETWEEN 5:00 AND 6:00 A.M. NATURALLY WITHOUT AN ALARM CLOCK

Once you start to go to bed at the right (that is, earlier) time, you'll naturally find it easier to wake up earlier, too. Embrace this, and once it becomes habit, try doing so without any alarm clock at all.

BE CAREFUL WITH SUPPLEMENTS AND MEDICINE

Magnesium and specialty supplements that have been

formulated for sleep are definitely worth experimenting with in the framework. But stay away from melatonin and other "natural" sleep aids, because after a while, the body becomes dependent on these and won't produce melatonin on its own. It's okay to take anything that won't stop natural cycles, though.

CLEAR YOUR MIND OF JUDGMENT

This isn't directly related to better sleep practices, but I think it's worth mentioning because it has the potential to also improve your sleep.

Nighttime can be the most anxiety-prone and stress-filled time of the day. In bed, it's not uncommon for our monkey brains—which thrive in our chaotic and performance-driven culture—to start moving one hundred miles per hour, replaying the happenings of the day, thinking about all that there is to do the next day, and/or beating ourselves up for all we failed to do. Meditation teaches us to take things as they come without judgment, so I recommend that when you go to sleep at night, you lay to rest the fears and ruminations from your day. They won't serve you now, so let them go.

I realize many people also experience moments of panic and fear in the middle of the night, often after they've been asleep for a few hours. If you find this is the case, realize that it's normal—our ancestors often did this to feed a fire for warmth during the night (mostly red and yellow spectrum light, by the way, not blue). But instead of resorting to using your phone or laptop during times of insomnia or anxiety, use it as an opportunity to practice meditation, or just take a few deep breaths. Focus on your breathing, be patient with yourself, and let the feelings wash away with every breath out. Treat your body with compassion during times of frustration, and you'll find it easier to let go of anxiety.

OPTIMIZING YOUR SLEEP ENVIRONMENT

The quality of your sleep depends on the nutritional choices you make as well as the choices you make about your sleeping environment. When you get these two components right, you'll be more likely to get the deep, restorative sleep your body craves, and wake up with a clear mind, ready to face the day.

Here are some basic guidelines to optimize your sleep environment:

- *Remember, your bedroom is a sacred space for sleeping and intimacy.* When your ancestors retired to sleep, they weren't lying there watching television, scrolling through their Instagram feed, or running through their schedule for the next day. That's why you need to make sure your bedroom is reserved for sleep and intimacy, and not television-watching, working, or anything else that could be considered a modern distraction. By simplifying your sleep environment, you'll calm your monkey brain and prepare it for stillness, quiet, and connecting with your partner. Remember, you're at the mercy of your subconscious at night, so optimize for activities that are calming and stress-relieving.

- *Replace your mattress.* You've probably heard how important it is to regularly replace your mattress (experts suggest you do so once every eight years), but this is something most people ignore. For some reason, a lot of people completely overlook the importance of maintaining an item where they'll spend one-third of their life. I ignored this notion, too—that is, until I went on a trip one week and slept better than I'd ever slept, on a brand new mattress in an RV. Right when I got back home, I replaced my mattress, and I urge you to do the same if you're having trouble sleeping. You'd be surprised how much an old mattress contributes to the quality of your sleep. Look for modern ones that are specifically designed for the type of sleeper you are (back, side sleeper, and so on). There are also many mattresses that are designed with materials that keep you cooler, and, as a result, more comfortable at night.
- *Invest in a high-quality pillow.* This is another dimen-

sion of the sleeping environment that gets ignored. Each person has different needs for their pillow, but, like a mattress, it's something you'll inevitably use every day. While the optimal sleep position is on your back, many people move to their side later, where the pillow becomes more important for the neck. Test a few pillows and start with high-quality ones that contain natural or low-allergen materials, or are designed to keep you cool. A good pillow doesn't need to be replaced very often and is maybe $100 to $150, far less expensive than a mattress, making this a good place to start with experimenting in your sleep space. Before you balk at the idea of dropping over $100 on a pillow, just think about it—how often will you replace your pillow? Probably not that often, which means $100 over time is a pretty low cost per use.

- *Keep your bedroom as dark as possible.* As I've mentioned, there's no need to have a television in your room or to be staring at your phone right before bed. I've got blackout blinds that don't let any light through, and I put a piece of tape over the light on my smoke detector or anything else that might have light directed directly at me. I actually travel with this tape, as well, because, for reasons I'll never understand, hotels place their smoke detectors right over their beds. The first time I noticed this was when I was experimenting with wearing blue-light-blocking glasses before sleep a few hours prior to bedtime.

When I took them off, I saw a light beaming down on my face from the smoke detector. This might seem like a small, silly thing, but any unnatural light is important to remove because your body was made to sleep mostly in the dark. Again, your ancestors weren't sleeping with smoke alarms above their beds. As for the moon and the stars, there is some dispute among scientists and researchers about these, but what's important to note is that they aren't blue light—they're on the orange and red spectrum.

TRACKING YOUR SLEEP AND CONTINUING YOUR JOURNEY

If you're going to experiment with optimizing your sleep, there's one piece of advice that's more important than any other: *don't overthink it*. Most of what we do during our waking hours—move our bodies, eat whole foods, avoid alcohol, take a few key supplements, and so on—has more potential to improve our sleep than the majority of crazy contraptions or devices that claim to enhance our sleep. One major exception: I do recommend wearing an Oura ring for tracking your sleep patterns and getting accurate data. That's because of all the sleep tests I've undertaken, it's the least invasive. Let's be honest: if you've got to wear a nose cannula or have fifteen to twenty-five diodes connected to your chest and body, wires dangling every which way, those tests might provide data, but they're in no way accurate representations of a normal night's sleep.

To keep things simple with sleep experiments, here are a few straightforward tips:

1. **Do proper intake at the start.** Before you can really analyze and compare anything, you need a decent baseline. That's why it's good to ask yourself the following questions before starting your sleep experiments:
   - What time do you go to sleep now?
   - What time do you wake up?
   - Do you wake during the night?
   - How do you feel when you wake up?
   - How do you feel when you check in with yourself throughout the day?
   - Do you struggle to focus, or have any other cognitive challenges that might be related to sleep? Feel free to add any other questions that you feel might be relevant for establishing a baseline profile of your sleep patterns—the answers will serve as the "before" to your after. And remember, if you track the answers to these questions at the start, you must ask yourself these same questions *throughout your experimentation*. This will allow you to track changes over time and across all variations of your experimentation.

2. **Don't make radical decisions based on one night of sleep.** One night's worth of sleep doesn't produce enough data about your sleep to reveal any significant patterns. If you're going to track and test your sleep, make sure you allow enough time to elapse so that you can observe and collect enough information. Tossing and turning one night isn't a pattern; it's an unfortunate event that may or may not be making much of an impact on your overall sleep quality. I recommend you observe your sleep behavior for a few weeks, perhaps a month, before analyzing the data. Otherwise, there's just not enough data to work with.

3. **Measure what really matters.** If you're going to measure sleep stages, I recommend focusing less on the specific time in each stage and focus instead on how you might be able to increase your deep sleep and cycling between stages.

4. **Figure out if you've got a sleep disorder.** If you think you've got an actual sleep disorder, experimenting might delay the resolution of your sleep problems or make them much more difficult to manage. I recommend figuring this out *before* doing a ton of experimentation, as there might be a more serious underlying issue. I would definitely consider in-depth, clinical testing—and I'd take the data very seriously. If you snore a lot or wake up gasping for air, get tested right away, as you might have sleep apnea. This means you actually stop breathing at times while

you sleep. Though some clinical sleeping problems like restless leg syndrome are bogus in my opinion, there are others that are serious and necessary to diagnose for the sake of your own health. If you think you've got a true medical sleep disorder, you'll most likely have to complete an at-home test along with an in-lab sleep study called a PSG (polysomnography). Interestingly, I wore my Oura ring while I was doing the most advanced clinical testing available (both at-home and in-lab) and my Oura ring data was very close to the data that clinical testing produced. It's much more comfortable sleeping with an Oura ring, too. If you want to measure quantitative sleep data, the Oura ring is what I recommend.

5. **Don't over-experiment.** Develop a few key hypotheses, and make minor adjustments based on patterns that emerge. If you've found something that works to produce better sleep, you don't need to continue testing every variable under the sun.

If you definitely don't have a sleep disorder, I recommend experimenting with other gadgets like blue-light-blocking glasses, which I mentioned earlier, especially if you spend much of your day in front of the computer. I've personally used them to block light throughout the night and other times when I've switched time zones and needed to trick my body a bit. You can also use PEMF (pulsed electromagnetic field therapy), which was developed by

NASA, as a sleep device to test in the framework. PEMF helps people get to sleep and stay asleep using pulsating magnetic fields that help the brain find its way into a state of deep rest. This, however, is also extremely expensive—usually about $500 to $1,500 per device.

Over the years, I've invested a ton of time and a lot of resources into experiments that would optimize my sleep. Hundreds of hours of sleep tests and tweaks with and without gadgets, both in my home and in sleep labs. But you don't have to do any of that. That's why I've limited this section to a few key ideas and tactics that provide better return on investment than others out there. That being said, if you're curious about something, I urge you to try it out. Just remember the Pareto principle, and why a small amount of targeted effort has the potential to influence most of your results.

But beyond the advice in this chapter, some of the most powerful factors in getting a good night's sleep revolve around the basics: moving your body during the day, eating whole foods, avoiding alcohol, and abstaining from eating within three hours of your bedtime. And while it might be uncomfortable and challenging to not stare at your phone before bed or to refrain from turning the television on to numb your mind, these small changes have potential for producing major magical moments. In time, you'll get used to it and finally be able to tap into the natural rhythm of your body. Push yourself and stick to your journey, and you'll likely wake up fully rested and ready to take on the day—just like when you were a child.

Dig deeper into the science of sleep at www.unstoppablebook.com/chapter13.

CHAPTER 14

EXERCISE, MOVEMENT, AND ALIGNMENT

When I was in my twenties and struggling with my weight and nutrition, I thought exercise was the answer. I'd hit the gym every single day for at least an hour—sometimes more—to sweat off the calories, and to absolve myself of the nutritional sins I thought I'd committed. In my thirties, I took up extreme endurance sports to allow myself to eat whatever I wanted, whenever I wanted. Even though it didn't help me keep weight off long-term, and left me with chronically painful knee problems, I believed in the power of exercise. And *lots* of it. But I wasn't alone. Everyone around me seemed to be obsessed with the gym, putting in their time each day to get healthier and fitter than ever before.

The only problem?

I was miserable. As I registered for one endurance competition after another, my muscles, bones, and joints ached. I was constantly hungry because of the number of calories I was burning, but I felt shame for eating as much as I did. My sleeping habits were awful, too. Not only did I not prioritize sleep back then, but I was also staying up late working each night because I had fewer hours during the day to get work done. I was stuck in a perpetual cycle of "doing," a form of inertia that kept me pushing through the frustration and the pain. And, you know what? I was praised for it. That's how powerful the myth of exercise is in our culture.

The thing is, many of us have been taught that exercise is half of what it takes to be healthy (the other half being diet). If someone is spending hours in the gym—"crushing" their personal fitness or whatever people are calling it these days—it's viewed as admirable. Enviable. Healthy. But in reality, it's not. Misery and pain don't equal health.

You may have picked up this book expecting a good chunk of the recommendations would be related to fitness and working out. After all, the myth of exercise is, as I mentioned, a powerful one—I was under its control for a frustrating fifteen years. But, these days, I can say from experience that I've completely transformed the way I think about exercise and understand its role in the journey to health and wellness. In the next few pages, I'll dive into exactly what that means and why it's highly likely that your current fitness routine is doing you more harm than good.

MISCONCEPTIONS

I'm certainly not saying that exercising isn't important. I still belong to a gym, and you'll see me there six days a week, practicing yoga, regularly lifting, and occasionally, in a spin class. But what I'm saying is that exercise has been framed incorrectly for a long time in our culture. Instead of thinking of exercise as moving your body and being active, we tend to conjure up notions of spending hours in the gym burning calories.

But I challenge you to abandon that harmful notion. In fact, I want you to think about exercise a different way. When you hear the word "exercise," I want you to think *movement*.

Why define exercise this way?

Because it has the potential to liberate you from outdated and/or ineffective forms of exercise that could be standing in the way of your health. I'm going to be looking at exercise through a lens that you probably haven't used before—and, hopefully, it'll actually make you *want* to exercise by removing what makes it feel like a burden. At the end of the day, exercise doesn't need to feel like this—it can and should be a source of personal satisfaction, social interaction, and connecting with nature. Use it to your advantage, not to your emotional and physical detriment.

So, what's the truth about exercise? Keep reading to find out.

THE TRUTH ABOUT EXERCISE

- *Exercise has little to do with burning calories.* One of the oldest and most prevalent myths is that exercise is all about burning calories. Yes, it's important to burn calories as humans, but you shouldn't be moving just to burn off your last meal. You should be moving—exercising—for the joy of being able to do so. Counting steps, counting calories, and all these different kinds of tracking disciplines only rob you of the joy you can experience when you're moving your body instead of punishing it with hours on an elliptical. Counting can be helpful if it leads to changes in behavior, but your number of steps, for example, really doesn't matter. Sometimes wearing my Oura ring helps to remind me to take the stairs every time I press the button for an elevator—and this is good because the ring reminds me to be active—but as far as changing my behavior, it does little. To keep things simple, focus instead on *moving when you can* throughout the day. For example, if you've got a meeting that's half of a mile away from your office, leave a little early and walk instead of catching an Uber. If you have a dentist appointment on the fifth floor, take the stairs instead of waiting for the elevator. These, again, are small changes that deliver huge rewards over time, especially when combined with the right diet. Notice that these kinds of "exercise" don't involve beating yourself to a pulp for two hours at the gym each day. Still not buying it?

Well, let me ask you a question: is it better to remain sedentary for most of the day, except for two grueling hours at the gym working out? Probably not. Try to think of incremental ways to move throughout the day and reduce the need for targeted sweat sessions that leave you wiped out.

· *Exercise has little to do with repetition.* Another misconception is that you need to do the same exercise every day in order to get in shape. A lot of people go to the gym each day and run or walk on the treadmill—nothing else. I did this for a long time too. Whenever I was calorie counting, I knew exactly how long I needed to run based on what I ate during the day or the night before. Whenever I was doing endurance sports, I was on a strict training schedule that required me to run outside each day, steadily increasing my mileage with time. But in both scenarios, I was putting my body through the exact same movements, and all that does is teach your body how to move the same muscles, over and over again. Truth be told, there should be diversity in your movement. Sure, it's important to have a routine, but not a routine that conditions your body to strengthen the same muscles every day. For example, I go to yoga at the same time in the morning, six days a week, but the flow is always different: it pushes my body in different ways, and the movement is always changing. I mostly do hot Vinyasa yoga, so it exercises my heart and builds strength, just like when I was running frequently. But, unlike running, the variation in movement uses different muscles and incorporates my entire body and mind. Sometimes I'll also lift weights before yoga or do a spin class at night. Diversity and enjoyment are crucial for staying healthy.

- *Exercise has little to do with "cardio."* I've heard the word "cardio" in the context of fitness with such frequency and passion that you'd think it had the ability to cure all the world's problems. But in reality, it doesn't. Don't ask me how the idea took hold—perhaps due to its association with burning calories—but the notion that cardio is more important than strength training is just plain wrong. You see, muscle burns more calories at rest than cardio, and also helps retain muscle mass and strength as we age. The human body, however, was designed to be a strong machine—it can move things, pick things up, and build things. As modern humans, we do less manual labor, sure, but our muscles were still made to be used. And, even when you're not actively using them, your muscles are burning calories without you even feeling it. So focus on diverse workouts that build your *strength*, and don't obsess as much over doing endless amounts of cardio. Bodyweight exercises, like push-ups and pull-ups, are also great if you have minimal equipment.

RECOMMENDATIONS FOR EXERCISING AND MOVING THE BODY

Heart health drives many people to exercise regularly. But unfortunately, the exercises that many rely on to stay healthy consist entirely of cardio routines. Whether you're doing hours on the elliptical or logging miles on a treadmill, or taking it to the extreme with the kind of endurance sports I participated in for years, you're putting yourself under unnecessary stress and strain without much benefit. After all, it's been proven that most, if not all, people's bodies have long-term damage[60] due to the intensity of endurance sports. In many cases, this has caused permanent tearing around the heart tissue.

---

60 "Can Too Much Extreme Exercise Damage Your Heart?" Cleveland Clinic, September 11, 2014, https://health.clevelandclinic.org/can-too-much-extreme-exercise-damage-your-heart/.

The truth is, human bodies aren't made for this kind of exercising. I no longer train for marathons or Ironman races like I used to. Instead, I get my heart rate up through other forms of movement that usually last no more than sixty to ninety minutes, like hot yoga, spin, or high-intensity interval training. There are obviously all kinds of different ways to work out that are extremely beneficial to the short-term and long-term health of your heart.

If you're looking for a means of measuring what's healthy or unhealthy when exercising your heart, the important thing to target is your heart rate variability (HRV). Your HRV measures the space between beats and your heart-rate recovery, which gauges how long it takes your heart to get back to a resting or normal heart rate after a high-intensity workout. Measurements like these are vastly more important than counting your steps or calories. Be careful, too, when looking at measurements like actual heart rate, because the reality is that heart rate differs from person to person. So, unless you've done heart-rate testing to find your intervals or levels, then I don't think that heart-rate variability and heart-rate recovery are useful. Any "averages" you find outside of your own data are just random estimates based on height and weight, which most likely won't be accurate for your own unique body. If you want to dig into these things, go for it. Perform some heart-rate testing. Find your thresholds.

But unless you're measuring the right metrics, don't pay attention to it.

Participating in endurance sports can damage your body permanently, but so can not doing anything with it at all. That's why I think it's unfortunate that so many of us spend the majority of our days sitting at desks.

We've gone from constantly being on our feet, running around outside, hunting and gathering, to sitting inside all day long under artificial light. It's an unnatural way of being human, and yet, many of us do it every day. If you're on your feet all day, then this might not apply to you, but if you work at a desk, you can strengthen your core through posture variation: invest in a standing desk, go on a walk, do a few push-ups after your conference call to get the blood flowing. Overall, just try to use your muscles throughout the day. Like I've said many times, small decisions add up to massive change over time. For example, I was experiencing a lot of back pain, so I asked my doctor what I could do to fix it. He suggested a number of different exercises, which didn't help at all. I finally invested in a standing desk that I could raise to any height, and my back pain decreased right away.

Another strategy that's effective for combating the fatigue and stiffness associated with desk work is something I call the 2:15 method. For every two hours I spend at my desk, I make sure I have fifteen minutes of movement *away* from it. This isn't only good for your body, but it's also good for your mind. Establishing routines like this can keep you in check whenever you're in over your head with work. When your day is crazy, your routine will make sure that the health of your body is prioritized, which will benefit your work. Having a routine is especially important while traveling. If, say, I'm traveling, I'll pull up a seven-minute workout app on my phone in the morning to get the blood flowing before the start of the day. There are also plenty of body-weight exercises that you can do during pauses throughout your day and many opportunities to move. Figure out when you'll get those fifteen-minute breaks I mentioned above and you'll start to build variation and healthy routines, even when you're away from home.

THERAPIES AND PRACTICES FOR OPTIMIZING BODY FUNCTION

Exercising and moving is great. They help with heart health and blood flow. They release good chemicals into the brain. They build muscle and help you to tap into how your body was made to operate. But there are a ton of other great types of practices that promote wellness within your body. Remember: how you feel is critical to how healthy your body is.

MASSAGE AND REALIGNMENT

One of my favorite go-to therapies and practices is massage. People have been getting massages for hundreds of thousands of years. And, in addition to feeling good, massage does amazing things like detoxify your body, realign your muscles, and target areas of pain and tightness. Like I said, it doesn't just feel good, it works. Regular massage can relieve problems caused by how you sit, or how you move. The problem with massage is that it's expensive and time-consuming, which is why a lot of people ignore it. However, I highly recommend prioritizing this and looking into what your insurance covers so that you can reduce the costs of massage and get the benefits.

If your insurance doesn't cover massage, or if it's just too expensive, try foam rolling. The foam roller is light, easy to travel with, and allows you to roll out your muscles anywhere and anytime you want. Best of all, you don't have to spend a ton of money to get the benefits of muscle realignment.

Egoscue, named after its inventor, Pete Egoscue, is another specific therapy in the area of alignment that focuses on your natural posture. By identifying imbalances you may have and working to realign them, you can avoid long-term problems. This kind of therapy is less about perfect alignment and more about personal alignment. A good Egoscue practitioner will spend the time studying how you stand or sit and will be able to tell you whether your left or right side is more dominant. The practitioner will then give you specific exercises that you can do to help your body get back to a more balanced position that will decrease long-term damage.

INFRARED LIGHT AND SAUNAS

Two more practices that have similar beneficial effects: infrared light exposure and spending time in the sauna. These are areas of heat variation or heat exposure, which help with numerous functions in the body. Exposure to infrared light is an especially important practice because most people don't get enough exposure to it during the day. Infrared light detoxifies your body and helps you sleep.

Because your body resets itself when exposed to extreme temperatures, sitting in a sauna that's 120 to 150 degrees (for short intervals) helps with detoxification, relaxation, and loosening your muscles. There are a number of internal mechanisms in your body that recover whenever these extreme exposures happen. And, to me, the best thing about both of these therapies and practices are the possibilities during the time you invest in these activities. A lot of times I listen to an audiobook, read, or watch something relaxing and/or useful on my phone. This is a space where you can do something to improve your mind while you're also helping your body.

COLD THERAPY

Your body was made to handle extreme differences in temperatures. When our ancestors' bodies were exposed to extreme cold, this activated important internal functions in order to prevent death. Cold therapy, as you might guess, simply involves extreme cold exposure. This is a practice that has been especially trendy and "hot" as of late (no pun intended), particularly in health and wellness circles.

The main benefit of cold therapy?

It increases *brown* fat, as opposed to *adipose* fat, in the body. Brown fat is actually the kind you want to have. It does a lot of beneficial things like boosting immunity and metabolism. We also know that cold therapy helps with muscle recovery. Think about the football player who's known to take an ice bath after a strenuous football game or basketball players who have ice packs on their legs on the bench. In both cases, cold temperatures are aiding in muscle recovery. Best of all, experimenting with cold therapy has no down side, as long as you're being smart and not doing ridiculous things like burning your skin with ice.

Here are some options for experimenting with cold therapy:

- *Take a cold shower.* This one's obvious: the easiest way to experiment with cold therapy is to simply take a cold shower. Start with thirty seconds of cold, then try to work your way up to two or three minutes by regularly doing this over time. Taking a cold shower for an extended period of time might feel uncomfortable at first, but just stick with it. Stand beneath the water and focus on your breathing. You'll be surprised by what your body can actually handle, following the initial shock of the coldness. Move your body around, and make sure that all of its parts are exposed to the cold, including your armpits, neck, back, and shoulders—areas that the water might not directly hit if you're just standing still. If that sounds too intimidating, start by taking your usual warm or hot shower, and end your shower with thirty seconds of cold. Although this is an area that's still being researched, there's no downside to experimenting with cold therapy, as long as you're careful with it. Many people believe that it leads to increased energy, heightened focus, and reduced stress levels.

· *Implement more variation in your showers.* If you find through experimentation that this therapy is beneficial, and you've increased the length of your cold shower to two or three minutes over time, you can take cold therapy to the next level by experimenting with extremes: switch between warm or hot water, and then make the water as cold as possible. This variation simulates what our ancestors likely experienced with the change of seasons—something that our bodies haven't really been exposed to in our increasingly temperature-controlled environments. Some suggest ten seconds of hot water followed by thirty seconds of cold water, repeated several times. Just experiment with it. There's no set way to go back and forth between these extreme temperatures. I usually just use this alternating strategy during the final two minutes of my shower or simply finish my shower with a couple minutes of cold water—it just depends on how much time I have.

- *Experiment with ice baths, cold compression, or cryotherapy.* Once you've conquered cold showers and varied extreme temperatures, it's time for the more dramatic stuff like ice baths, cold compression, and cryotherapy. All of these involve the exposure to freezing or near-freezing temperatures. I find cold compression to be especially interesting. Ice baths are more daunting and difficult, requiring you to have a very expensive cold-exposure tub in your house or your gym. Intense cold therapy has been popularized by Wim Hof, who combines cold therapy with breath work. Known as the "Iceman," he has done all kinds of things with cold exposure, like climbing the highest mountains in the world only wearing shorts, or swimming underneath ice for sixty-six meters. Though I've been to several Wim Hof events and have found them to be beneficial, I strongly urge you to start by taking a cold shower, see if it works for you, and then continue your experimentation from there.

PEMF

When you first start looking into PEMF (pulsed electromagnetic field) therapy, you'll be tempted to think that it's a scam. And I totally get it—it sounds ridiculous. But it's not. It was actually developed by NASA and has been studied extensively in the medical field for pain relief, muscle issues, sleep, and all sorts of other things. PEMF uses bursts of electromagnetic radiation to heal damaged tissues and bone, or relieve pain. These frequencies pulse similarly to how the brain functions during a sleep state.

PEMF is interesting because it's becoming more accessible through the production of mobile units, which are expensive but growing increasingly cheaper over time. These mobile units used to be $10,000, and now you can find a device from anywhere between $600 and $5,000. It's definitely an investment, but the good thing about it is that it can be used for a variety of different things, whether it's movement, alignment function, pain, or sleep challenges. A PEMF unit is definitely a good long-term investment.

KEY TAKEAWAYS

If going to the gym feels like you're "putting in your time" each day, then you're not exercising, you're just punishing yourself. It may sound dramatic, but that's because I feel strongly that moving your body is a gift that should be celebrated. Getting stronger and more flexible should be a great opportunity to connect with yourself and others around you. And whatever you do, whether it's yoga, going for a run, dancing, whatever, make sure it's joyful.

In employing some of the strategies, practices, and therapies I've mentioned in this chapter, your body will begin to feel better *and* operate more efficiently. A lot of people mistakenly think their bodies have to be sore or aching all of the time for exercise and movement to be beneficial, but I fear that we're actually causing more long-term damage to our bodies by inflicting this pain. Be smart and intentional, not reckless. Remember the myths that I've already discussed. In this area of your life, ask yourself the questions:

- Why are you doing what you're doing?
- Is it rooted in research?
- Is it rooted in personal experimentation?

Or are you just doing what I did for so long in my life, simply following what popular culture is telling you to do?

Get access to scientific research about exercise, cold therapy, and more at www.unstoppablebook.com/chapter14.

CHAPTER 15

MICRO-OPTIMIZATIONS THAT MAKE A DIFFERENCE

Optimizing your nutrition, sleep, and exercise has the potential to produce *huge* changes in your life. After obsessively researching these areas as well as using my own body to experiment, I've seen the proof firsthand. And while the core components of this book have been focused on broader optimizations designed to make you unstoppable, this chapter will focus specifically on what I call *micro-optimizations*. While they cover many parts of your life—from your work environment and daily routine to techniques that fuel productivity and focus—they'll be united by one theme: they're all small changes that can make a big difference in the long run.

Micro-optimizations like the ones I'm about to share emerged as I used this framework over time. Since they're my own personal discoveries, I don't expect them all to work for you. But they can still be a great catalyst for you to discover your own micro-optimizations outside the confines of the larger experimentation you'll be doing.

So let's dig in.

MICRO-OPTIMIZATIONS

For thousands of years, our ancestors were leading highly active lifestyles, rising with the sun, sleeping at nightfall, and eating whole foods they were able to hunt or gather. In stark contrast to modern life, there were no desk jobs, no staring at computer screens, and certainly no processed foods to snack on. And our ancestors were better off for it.

Today, our sedentary lifestyles and poisoned food supply have sent our bodies into revolt. Rising rates of obesity, stress, chronic disease, and a host of other issues are on the rise. Even though we live in a time of rapid technological innovation, we fail to innovate the way we treat these mounting medical issues so that people can lead happier and healthier lives.

I'm certainly not saying we need to go back to the past.

I love technology and the conveniences it affords. But I am saying that there are a number of ways we can alter the modern world to reflect the way our ancestors lived and, in the process, optimize our own lives.

For example, although the majority of us work in offices and will never have the same amount of exposure to the outdoors as our ancestors did, it's still important to connect with nature on a regular basis. When we unplug and push away from our desks—and our screens—we see a huge potential for shifts in stress levels, mood, and more. And this is just one example—there are many, many more. In this chapter, I'm going to focus on outlining the small changes—or *micro-optimizations*—we can make in order to influence our lives, all based on my own experiences or the conversations I've had with countless wellness experts, medical professionals, and even other entrepreneurs.

OPTIMIZING YOUR WORK ENVIRONMENT AND PHYSICAL WORKSPACES

Headaches, back pain, lack of focus, distraction, low productivity, and eyestrain are symptoms of the modern workplace. Though some of you may recognize them as signs of a hard day's work, they're actually warning signs from your body that something isn't right.

You see, many—if not all—of the problems I listed above

are caused by the modern workplace and the tools that we use there. For example, many offices limit natural light and expose us to a ton of blue light, overstimulating our senses and sometimes causing heaviness in our eyes that can make it difficult to sleep. Making some simple adjustments in this area of your life could have multiple benefits, helping you to focus later in the workday, and sleep better when you go to bed. Here's a short list of micro-optimizations I've experimented with and find valuable.

Turn off fluorescent lights. Fluorescent lights emit blue light, just like your computer and phone screens, which has been shown to decrease melatonin production and cause sleep disturbances.[61] If you have these in your office, try turning them off for a few hours a day. I find turning them off in the afternoon is most beneficial as I begin to transition from the workday into the evening.

Open the blinds. Natural light is good light. If you can move your desk closer to a source of natural light, do it. If you can't, make sure that natural light isn't obstructed in any way.

Stand up and move around. Humans weren't meant

---

61   Victoria L. Dunckley, "Why CFL's Aren't Such a Bright Idea," *Psychology Today*, September 15, 2014, https://www.psychologytoday.com/us/blog/mental-wealth/201409/why-cfls-arent-such-bright-idea.

to sit for eight hours a day. But they weren't necessarily meant to do the opposite—stand for hours on end—either. So do yourself a favor and do *both*, with a healthy dose of other movements and stretches in between, too.

Get a red light or sunlamp. Although red light is often associated with treating wrinkles and boosting collagen production, it may also have the potential to increase energy, or at least counteract the light sources in most office environments. In addition, a sunlamp may provide some reprieve from workplaces starved for natural light.

Install f.lux or Iris Pro. Programs like f.lux and Iris Pro automatically adjust your screens to match the time of day and the room that you're in to allow for more red light to be emitted. Either program can be installed on your laptop or mobile device.

Take a walk. Whatever you do, *never* sit at your desk or remain inside for the entire day. By taking a quick walk outside, you get a trio of benefits: natural light, movement, and fresh air. Nothing better than that.

Okay, so we've covered all of the small adjustments you can make to feel better and tweak your workplace environment. But what everyone's really after at work is *productivity*. That's why the next few optimizations can be combined with everything I mentioned above in order to maximize productivity while improving your health:

- *Put a process in place.* If you're struggling to optimize your productivity and haven't read *Getting Things Done* by David Allen, stop what you're doing and get yourself a copy now. This book is a classic for both productivity and process. At a high level, Allen discusses the importance of creating lists and targeting the three most important tasks to get done each day. If you accomplish your three most important tasks, then formulate another list with the next three most important tasks. This simple strategy will help your brain to focus, and simply take one step after another throughout the day so that it doesn't get overwhelmed. Your to-do list should be realistic, or else it defeats the purpose of a to-do list.

- *Delegate.* Learning to delegate is a skill that you can develop both intellectually and emotionally. True delegation is more than just enlisting someone else's help; it's having the emotional capacity to truly let go of the responsibility once it's been delegated. You don't get the benefits of delegation if you hand off a project to someone yet continue to micromanage it. You need to be able to actually let go. And there are many benefits to be had: you can get more done, feel less stressed, and empower other people to move a project forward. As an entrepreneur, I struggled with delegation for years. I found it extremely difficult to ask others for help, and even when I did, I never truly let go of the task because I thought I could get it done better or faster. In the beginning of running my business, this may have been true. But once I made a practice of hiring smarter and more specialized people, I finally learned to let go. What's more, the company evolved faster than it would have if I continued to be a bottleneck. Delegation also freed me up to do more valuable work that was more in line with my primary skillset, and also positioned others to take more ownership of the company's success.

- *Get an assistant or virtual assistant.* If you're establishing a process, prioritizing, creating a to-do list, and delegating, then a virtual assistant (or VA) can help you to stay on track and help you to feel like you have your day under control. My VA helps with lots of personal and household tasks, making appointments, dealing with vendors, checking prices, researching, setting up appointments, following up on bills, or other things that should've gotten done by others. Once you get good at this, you'll start to look for more valuable tasks for your assistant to complete.

- *Beware of tool lusting.* Tech companies are always releasing new products with all sorts of promises attached to them, swearing that they'll benefit your life or revolutionize your workplace. Don't get hung up on all the different gadgets and gizmos out there.

Stick to your routine and what works for you. If writing out your to-do list each morning with pen and paper works for you, stick to it. Formulate a clear strategy with what you have and execute it. I've seen far too many people complicate their lives due to having too many tools to manage. Keep it simple.

- *Turn off ALL notifications on your phone and computer.* This is simple, but it's so difficult for people to do because they either have a fear of missing out, or actually *like* to be distracted throughout the day. My phone is always on silent. My computer doesn't ding or even receive a pop-up window when I receive an email. The only thing that pops up on any of my devices are calendar notifications—necessary interruptions to remind me of meetings. These calendar notifications actually free me to get lost and absorbed in my work because I know that I can focus fully on the task at hand and will be reminded by my calendar whenever I need to move on to a meeting or other obligation. Eliminate all distractions that aren't related to work.

- *Put everything in your calendar.* For me, if it's not in the calendar, it doesn't happen. This also means scheduling fitness or meditation time, scheduling learning or reading, or even blocks of undistracted time to think and work. Just like routine, this is one of the most liberating things you can do. Be greedy and strict about your time. Your calendar helps you to create boundaries, which free you up in the areas that are most important to you. For example, I won't take meetings or calls during the time I have scheduled for yoga.

- *Use email to your advantage.* Learn how to effectively manage your emails. Whenever I get an automated email from someone about not answering their emails at a certain time of day, it drives me nuts. Only responding to emails once or twice a day is stupid and not productive. I can get more done, far faster, with far more people by effectively managing my emails and delegating than some people do in endless meetings and calls. In fact, I'd take an email over a phone call any day. Whereas some meetings can go on forever with endless small talk and pointless conversation, email forces you to get to the point. It's the easiest way in our culture to show availability and accessibility. It's the easiest way to optimize people's time. People don't want to do business or work with someone who isn't available and accessible. Never go more than twenty-four hours without responding to an email. I'm a big believer in Inbox Zero, the approach to email management that aims to keep the personal inbox empty. This is worth doing since much of business revolves around email. It'll clear your mind, let others know they can count on you, and force both task lists and delegation.

OPTIMIZING YOUR HOME ENVIRONMENT
THROUGH PERSONAL CARE AND HYGIENE

Your skin, mouth, eyes, and ears are like sponges, absorbing the elements that make up your home environment. If you fill this environment with chemicals and things that harm you, your body will absorb them just like it does the nutrients in the food you eat.

I know a lot of people who buy high-quality foods they've researched extensively for their own nutrition, but then buy low-quality personal care products with all kinds of chemicals in them. Be aware of the products you use. Some of these things are just as important as what you're putting into your stomach. Challenge your preconceived notions: don't ever assume that something's okay to purchase just because that's what you've always purchased, or that's what you grew up with.

Here are some of the main products in your physical environment that are worth investigating:

- *Deodorant.* Deodorant sticks contain ingredients that help manage underarm odor. But deodorant *and* antiperspirant products contain ingredients that manage odor and a chemical, aluminum, that prevents you from sweating altogether. By plugging sweat ducts, aluminum blocks wetness, leaving you "dry" all day. While this may seem like a good outcome, applying chemicals to this very sensitive area of the body is a risky proposition. Due to the presence of both sweat ducts and hair follicles, your underarm area is essentially a gateway to your body—what you apply to it is rapidly absorbed into your tissue and bloodstream. That's why you need to pay attention to the ingredients in these products. Aluminum, specifically, has been linked to breast and other cancers in the past, but research has been inconclusive.[62] Since the science still doesn't indicate a causal link, it's tough to say for sure if aluminum causes cancer, but why risk it? Just avoid these products entirely.

- ○ Remember, the body needs to sweat—it's part of how it takes care of itself. Don't prevent your body from doing what it naturally does. I know that it's not accepted in our culture to walk around with body odor or a smelly shirt, but there are natural deodorants that are much healthier and still very effective. I personally like crystal-based deodorants because they are 100 percent natural, composed of hard crystal or filtered water with crystal mineral in it. No irritation. No chemicals. And, whereas most deodorants that we buy *hide* body odor, this kind of deodorant will *prevent*

---

62 "Antiperspirants/Deodorants and Breast Cancer," National Cancer Institute, last modified August 9, 2016, https://www.cancer.gov/about-cancer/causes-prevention/risk/myths/antiperspirants-fact-sheet.

body odor. There are plenty of other options, too. Just do your research.

- *Oral care.* This area of optimization becomes much easier once you've cut out sugar and are following a low-carb diet, as sugar and carbs have a deleterious impact on oral health. But in addition to following the nutrition guidelines in this book, I'd strongly urge you to consider taking a look at both your toothbrush and toothpaste.

  - Toothbrush. You've probably heard that your toothbrush is extremely important—and that's definitely true. But you don't need to spend hundreds of dollars on electric toothbrushes to care for your teeth. I've a middle-of-the-line electric toothbrush that costs forty-five dollars and comes with new brush heads that last me through the year, and I can travel with it. Something like this will get you 80 percent to 90 percent of the way there. You don't need crazy spinning heads. You need small vibrations, guiding pulses, and a timer to make sure you are brushing for two minutes straight. This all goes back to minimal effort for maximum return. Two little changes—small vibrations and two straight minutes of brushing, when most people only brush for thirty seconds to one minute at the most—can make a big difference.

  - Toothpaste. Before you buy a toothpaste emblazoned with the word "natural" on it, take a closer look at the list of ingredients. There are some popular brands out there that are very misleading—they call their product "natural" when it's anything but that. In fact, many of these are actually filled with xylitol and fluoride, which should be avoided. Just like with other cosmetic and hygiene products, you should aim for as few ingredients as possible in your toothpaste. Fluoride has mostly been put into things, like toothpaste and our water supply, to compensate for our population's mass consumption of sugar. Like sugar, fluoride is a billion-dollar industry. But there's never a need to consume it. Think back to how the dentist puts fluoride on your teeth and reminds you not to swallow it—it's not good for you. Yet we do just that with toothpaste and water every single day, morning and night.

- Fillings. Investigate whether or not your fillings are composed of mercury. Do some research. Ask your dentist. There are a number of personal testimonies out there about how mercury from fillings has leaked into people's bodies from their teeth. Some have fixed significant medical issues that have plagued them for years—all from removing the mercury in their fillings.

- *Soap and shampoo.* Like toothpaste and deodorant, when it comes to soap and shampoo, you want to have as few ingredients as possible. I want to know what all the ingredients in my soap and shampoo are—I should be able to recognize their names. If there are a bunch of ingredients in your soaps that you cannot pronounce, that probably means there are a ton of chemicals, too. So do a little bit of legwork to find higher-quality, simpler shampoos and soaps. The nice thing is that today, there are a ton of options out there for natural soap and shampoo products. In the past they used to be hard to find; they're now all over the internet, and can be purchased in bulk to save money. Another added benefit to these products? They're gentler on the environment than mainstream products filled with chemicals.

- *Bathroom care.* The subject that no one likes to talk about is bowel movements—also known colloquially as pooping. But pooping is obviously vitally important. It's an instant indicator of health and wellness. It's silly to me that people are so afraid to talk about this topic when it's one of the most natural things that humans do, and provides instant insight into your own health, especially as you are experimenting within the framework. Do your homework and look into what different colors and forms of your poop tell you about your own nutrition. You need to know what's happening to your body and be unafraid to talk about it. In fact, if you're eating a good diet, then, as disgusting as this might sound, there should be no need for toilet paper. The reasons our ancestors didn't have to even think about toilet paper is because they weren't consuming the same processed and sugar-based foods that we eat today. Though I'm sure they experienced days where their stomachs were upset because of, say, bacteria in the water they drank or meat that they ate, they were also probably having natural poops because the foods they were consuming were part of their environment. Going back to evolution, one of the simple tools that I recommend for anyone and everyone is a Squatty Potty. This puts you in a natural squatting position that replicates what humans did before they had invented toilets, once again tapping into your own evolution and ancestry. It puts you into an optimal position for bowel evacuation. Use a Squatty Potty and you'll feel better throughout the day because you'll eliminate more from within you during your time in the bathroom. Lastly, I recommend having baby wipes in the bathroom. The idea of scraping paper against your butt doesn't make a lot of sense. But humans have had to do it because, frankly, their poops got messier because their diets became horrific. Follow the suggestions in this book, and your poops will become cleaner. If you don't have a bidet, then baby wipes will help your skin to feel better after pooping and, frankly, leave you much cleaner. I now travel with baby wipes and have them in both my suitcase and backpack.

- *Water sources.* Water is obviously essential to human survival. And, if you're following the nutrition and diet suggestions in this book, you'll find that it's even more important because of the role it plays in propelling your Unstoppable Lifestyle.
- Problem is, most people's water contains additives like fluoride and chlorine, along with many other chemicals, even in municipal or city water supplies. Some of the chemicals that have been added are necessary to prevent the water from accruing residue through pipes, but fluoride has been added to counteract the massive quantity of sugars present in our diet. There's no real reason fluoride would need to be added if we substantially decreased our consumption of sugar. Most people just assume that if they're drinking lots of water, that's a good thing, and *it is*—but your drinking habits can be optimized by installing a home filtration system. Be careful: a lot of filters that are sold today won't remove the chemicals that we're trying to remove. A home filtration system for your entire house might be pricey, but to me, it's well worth it considering the importance of water and the amount of water that you should be drinking. Remember, too, that you consume water in a number of different ways, whether it's cooking or bathing. I also invest in a local tap or under-counter filtration, preferably not reverse osmosis, so that I don't have to add mineralization back into the water

I drink. I can drink water right out of this tap and have the confidence that it has been optimized.

KEY TAKEAWAYS

Micro-optimizations like the ones we've covered in this chapter have the potential to make a massive difference in your health, productivity, and quality of life. From becoming more cognizant of the ingredients in your household products to cutting down on practices that put us at risk for disease, there are a ton of areas to focus your efforts. But don't be overwhelmed by all that can be optimized—instead, think of it as opportunity, and prioritize based on what's easiest for you to accomplish.

Another helpful way to look at micro-optimizations is as a starting point for bigger changes in your life. I know not everyone is going to be interested in starting some of the larger experiments we've discussed in this book, so the small changes I've listed above are a great way to get started with experimentation and graduate to some of the bigger changes around fuel, sleep, and exercise. That's what's helpful about the Unstoppable Lifestyle—you can begin anywhere.

For more on micro-optimizations, head to www.unstoppablebook.com/chapter15.

CHAPTER 16

MINDFULNESS PRACTICES

In mindfulness one is not only restful and happy, but alert and awake. Meditation is not evasion; it is a serene encounter with reality.

—THICH NHAT HANH

We live in a chaotic world. We lead busy lives, raise over-scheduled kids, and get praised for burning the candle at both ends. There's not much in our modern way of life that encourages us to live in the present moment and to encounter reality with the serenity Thich Nhat Hanh, a Buddhist monk, describes. But there's evidence we need to embrace mindfulness to lead fuller lives and make smarter decisions about the food we eat, and how we interact with friends and family.

Back when I was struggling with my weight and nutrition in my twenties and early thirties, I knew nothing of the practice of mindfulness. I'd inhale terrible foods, exercise relentlessly, get inadequate sleep, and wonder why I always felt like I was chasing some relentless and formless goal. It wasn't until I stepped foot in my first yoga class that I became acquainted with the idea of mindfulness that we'll discuss here—a practice of training your mind, and, by extension, your body.

In life, you often don't realize how much you need something until you try it. When I began to practice yoga regularly, I realized how chaotic and cluttered my mind was whenever I didn't practice yoga. Yoga had a way of helping me to see reality more clearly, and not put so much pressure on myself. Had I practiced mindfulness earlier on in my journey, when my health and wellness journey was marked by guilt and shame, I probably could've stopped self-judgment in its tracks. Nevertheless, I'm glad I discovered it at all, because it's changed my life. Below are seven principles from yoga teacher training that you should consider while on your journey. I not only apply these to my yoga practice, but try to implement them in every area of my life:

· You are exactly where you need to be.
· Fear and pain are life's greatest teachers.
· Laughter and play are the fountains of youth.

- Exercise and rest are essential to vibrant health.
- Intimacy and touch are basic human needs.
- Everything is impermanent.
- Everything is connected.

There are an endless number of mindfulness practices, but in this chapter, I'll be exploring the main ones that are easy to integrate into your life. Whether it's meditation, breathing, mindfulness, or yoga, each has been proven to lower stress, blood pressure, and heart rate, as well as increase concentration and productivity, presence, gratitude, and patience. Many people who have practiced this have used it successfully in managing anxiety and depression. What's more, some studies indicate that mindfulness practices may lower inflammation in the body—one of the main causes of heart disease, certain forms of diabetes, and chronic disease. They're also useful in dealing with mental and nervous system issues, depression, and post-traumatic stress disorder (PTSD).

You don't have to become a monk to practice mindfulness. You don't have to meditate for five hours a day. Instead, start simply: begin by meditating for one minute a day (really, this can be as simple as sitting still with your eyes closed for one minute) or focusing on your breath for two minutes a day or by attending yoga class. If it's too scary or difficult to think about entering into stillness and silence with your eyes closed, just try focusing on your breathing.

This is a good starting point for mindfulness: focusing on your breath, inhaling deeply through your nose, and feeling your belly contract and then fully expand with your breath. So many mindfulness practices get us back to the essentiality of breath, which is important because so many of us live our lives forgetting to take full and deep breaths. This kind of intentional breathing and breathing correctly—both of which I'll discuss at the end of this chapter—can make a really big difference in your life.

When I began to practice mindfulness regularly, I noticed big changes—and so did the people around me. People at work told me I seemed more patient. My girlfriend started telling me that I was more relaxed at home. When I began to research these outcomes, I uncovered studies that showed that meditation and mindfulness practices could have an impact in as little as five to ten minutes of your time a day. If you're curious about this practice and want to take this to the next level, go for it. There are retreats like Vipassana Retreats, and many others, that provide an immersive experience that deepens your practice. I'd love to join one of these types of experiences, but to be honest, I'm not there yet. I need to continue my practice and prepare for when I can be still with myself and make that type of investment. Remember, there's no rush when it comes to yoga, meditation, and mindfulness. Everyone's path is different. But if it interests you and you're ready to make the commitment, see where it leads you. Even if you're unable to attend a retreat, focusing on stillness and breath for five to ten minutes a day might be the easiest discipline you can adopt to lower stress levels and be more present in life.

What's even more wonderful about these mindfulness practices is that there's no downside to trying them. Their whole purpose is to serve as an ongoing practice that guides you to becoming more fully present in your life, which can lead to better relationships, an increased ability to focus, increased satisfaction after meals, and a host of other positive things.

YOGA

Yoga helped me to realize that mindfulness was the missing link in my life—it was the glue that held all of the different aspects of my world together. It simultaneously accomplished three things for me:

- *Physical strength.* The more active yoga, like hot Vinyasa flow, pushed me on a more holistic physical level than endurance sports had ever done. Due to the variation, it made me move differently, discover feelings within my muscles I used to ignore, and do things with my body that I never imagined possible. It also created a never-ending journey. Each step forward that I took in a single pose always opened another door, be it as simple as touching my toes for the first time or something as scary as attempting a handstand.

- *Social connection.* Yoga gave me a community and helped me to connect with people in a different way. No matter how challenging or grueling a class was, you knew that you were pushing yourself alongside others in a safe space where there was no room for judgment or criticism.
- *Spiritual awareness.* I've never been a religious person, but, for lack of a better term, yoga moved me spiritually, affecting me on a deep, personal level because of the practice of mindfulness. I found myself to be more compassionate at home and less judgmental of others out in public. And I became more aware of my own self-judgment and self-criticism.

I've shared my experiences with yoga first because it's effective on so many different levels that are essential to our health and well-being as humans. There are multiple types of yoga, but the highest return, for me, are the more active types that get your heart rate up and cause you to sweat, like Vinyasa, Power Yoga, Ashtanga, Core Power, Life Power, or similar. These kinds of yoga are rooted in the traditions of Ashtanga yoga.

My personal favorite is hot Vinyasa flow, and specifically Life Power, which is practiced in a heated room. Designed for detoxification, Life Power is less about flexibility and more about your active (or yang) poses, breathing, and linking breath with movement to find "seats" or poses for meditation. The class that I attend is also unique in the sense that the instructor guides you through a variety of different flows, and then, once he or she feels like those in the room understand the flow, lets you flow both at your own pace and taking your own journey. Throughout this class, you may add or subtract from the poses to find what's right for you and your body. I like this because I'm forced to focus on my own flow and remember the next pose. It's like remembering a dance, and the movement and focus helps me to be more present. This helps me get out of my head, where I tend to focus on the past or the future. I currently practice this kind of yoga six times a week.

If mindfulness is new to you as a concept and practice, another reason for trying yoga first is because it's all about movement, with the added benefit of building strength, raising your heart rate, and all the physical benefits you get along with this practice. In a busy society like ours, yoga can be a much easier transition into mindfulness compared with sitting still and meditating. I also think it's easier to walk into a yoga studio with anywhere between fifteen and fifty people than it is to attend a meditation class. This doesn't mean you can't work up to something like that over time. But one of the things I like most about yoga is that it's all about nonjudgment, for both yourself and others. The only important things are to focus on your own breath and challenge yourself to find your edge, whatever that means to you.

MEDITATION

Meditation is about freeing your mind and gently dismissing the things that naturally pop into your monkey brain. Don't misunderstand meditation by thinking that you have to think about nothing—that's almost impossible. It's more about being present in the current moment, which will, naturally, help you to think about less. The key to meditation is just accepting what passes through your mind, without judgment, as thoughts come and go. Accepting this simple fact will help you to bring more enjoyment into meditation and cultivate less self-judgment when you find it's difficult to quiet your mind.

So, what's the *goal* of meditation?

What I'm about to say is often very difficult for the Western mind to comprehend: meditation isn't something you *accomplish*. There are no "goals" associated with it. It's something to practice. Sometimes it'll feel pointless. Sometimes it might feel profound. It doesn't matter. There's no rating system and no judgment with meditation. The point is to feel, be present, and slow down. Once you accept there's no terminus in meditation, you'll start to see how powerful a practice it is.

A good starting point for meditation is to sit in stillness, silence, and solitude for one minute a day. Focus on your breath. Whatever thoughts arise, simply let them pass. Don't cling to them. Don't try to work anything out. *Just be.* The same goes for physical feelings: experience them, acknowledge them, and let them pass. From there, work your way up to five minutes. Then, if you want, slowly get up to fifteen minutes or twenty minutes. The data is clear that meditating for even a minute or two has almost all the benefits of longer meditation—once again, very little investment of time for a very substantial return.

There are many types of meditation, but I've only included the five main ones with descriptions that'll give you several good starting points. Experiment with each area and find what you like best. See what's most beneficial to your mind and personality, whether that's meditation that's guided by music, silent meditation, or meditation that moves through the entire body and catalogues different sensations. If you've never tried meditation, consider this the start of your personal journey.

- *Vipassana.* A traditional Buddhist type of meditation that's very much about awareness of your breath, Vipassana is translated, "To see things as they really are." The general way of practicing this is to tune into the feeling of your breath—noticing how it moves in and out of your nose. Maybe it's just noticing your breath on your top lip as it goes through your nostrils. Maybe it's simply noticing the warmth of the air coming out of your nose. Whatever rises into your mind regarding your breath, intensely focus on that specific thing. Again, this is a technique that brings focus to the current moment.

- *Zen.* This is similar to Vipassana and also comes from the Buddhist tradition, but this practice incorporates both your breath *and* thoughts. The goal is to bring awareness to your breath as you observe the thoughts and experiences that pass through your mind and body. Maybe it's an itch that you have on your toe that rises to the forefront of your mind. Instead of doing anything about it, simply let that thought pass and refrain from scratching your toe. Maybe an idea about something on your to-do list rises to the forefront of your mind. Don't stress over it, simply let it pass. There are other techniques where you move your focus toward sensations up and down your body or simply gain awareness of different feelings in the body or the happenings around you. It's all about observing—nonjudgmentally—the thoughts and experiences in the present moment and letting them pass over you.

- *Loving-kindness.* Though this kind of meditation has

just recently gained popularity, it comes from an old tradition within Buddhism known as Mettā meditation. The focal point of this practice is to think about unconditional love, kindness, and friendliness, whether that's giving gratitude to those whom you crossed paths with that day, or to those in your life whom you love and who love you, or to the other things in your life that stir joy within you. It's all about focus, and, in this case, intentionally positioning your mind—which tends to focus on the negative parts of life—to dwell upon positivity so that it leads to a posture of gratitude.

- *Transcendental.* This is a mantra-based meditation technique where you bring your focus to a mantra, and, no matter what arises in your mind, you keep focusing your attention on the mantra you've chosen. There are far deeper levels to this, but it's not my area of expertise. I'd recommend finding an instructor to guide you through the process to get the most out of this kind of meditation. This is very popular in India, but isn't as popular in the United States.

- *Kundalini.* This kind of meditation is all about tapping into different energy spaces in the body, located at the base of the spine. Once again, to really do this right, it requires training or instruction. Chakra is similar to Kundalini, targeting different energy centers in the body and accessing them through the mind.

There are also a number of apps that can help you to navigate meditation, along with plenty of guided meditations available on the internet. One thing to be aware of, however, is that some of these apps allow you to track the days you meditated, which can quickly become as pointless as tracking your steps or counting calories. Build meditation into your routine, but don't let it become something that you set out to "check off" your to-do list. That defeats the purpose of meditation. Also, remember not to be scared or intimidated. Meditation can be as simple as closing your eyes and sitting for a few minutes and focusing on your breath. There's no special mat or specific way to sit. You can even sit in a chair if it's more comfortable.

Meditation is a powerful tool that can have lasting impact on so many areas of your health. There's even some very interesting and emergent technology being developed that uses EEG and other tools to provide feedback during meditation. I don't think that these tools are reliable yet on a broad scale, but it's something to keep an eye on. It's possible in the future that these tracking devices will be able help people to discover certain feedback loops in their minds while meditating, and provide them with data regarding the origin of certain blockages in their minds. These blockages could explain why some people have the ability to be more "present" than others. But, this is very, very far off in the future.

At the end of the day, to truly benefit from practicing mindfulness, you must commit to it and build it into your routine. This is about you and what's best for you. Enter into it and let your mind be changed by it. You'll find yourself becoming more aware, present, grateful, centered, and compassionate.

BREATHING

Most of us have forgotten how to breathe. That's because we take breathing for granted. But focusing on our breath is actually critically important for our well-being and gets us back in touch with who we are.

The breath is one of the most interesting things about our bodies, as it can be both *unintentional* (automatically happening or involuntary), and *intentional* (controlled, changed, held). The best starting point for breathing is to focus on what a full and deep breath really is: allow the belly and lungs to expand in all directions with breath—into your sides, your chest, your back—followed by a deep and full exhalation, letting the body remove all the CO_2. You can do this by breathing in through the nose and out through the nose—controlled, intentional, and strong—or in through the nose, and out through the mouth. Whatever feels best for you. Many people have never done this or haven't done it in years. Do this four or five times. Try it for a few minutes. How do you feel afterward? More centered or less centered? What's different within you? You'll find each time that focusing on deep breathing will have a way of getting you back into the present moment and quieting your mind.

Breathing is the cornerstone for all meditative practice. Mindfulness is about breath. There are, however, specific types of breathing, or "breath work," that are worth exploring so that you can incorporate them throughout the hectic pace of your day, and in your meditation practice of choice—though it's important to know that each of them can be taken significantly deeper. These different breathing techniques will help you to get recentered and back into a state of peace and focus, but they're not an exhaustive list.

TYPES OF BREATHING

- *Box breathing.* This is also known as intentional deep breathing, and it's a very simple technique. Start by exhaling slowly and fully. Then inhale through your nose for four seconds, and, at the top of your inhalation, hold your breath for four seconds. Exhale through your mouth for four seconds, and then, at the bottom of your exhalation, hold your breath for four seconds. Then repeat the process. If you repeat this several times, you'll begin to realize how amazing it feels. Many actually start to feel as if they're high.

That's because when most people breathe normally, without thinking, they don't allow all the CO_2 to exit from their bodies because they're not fully pulling in all of the possible oxygen into their lungs. Box breathing gets you back to optimizing your breath. I often practice box breathing while sitting on a train or on a bus, or in my office, if I need a little break from work. It's very practical and many people find it to be extremely calming.

- *Buteyko.* This breathing method, formulated by a Ukrainian doctor named Konstantin Buteyko, was made popular beginning in the 1950s. Although there are many variations, the original version is fairly simple: take a small breath in, followed by a small breath out, then hold your breath for five seconds, and then relax for one minute. This should be repeated at least six times, preferably more. The goal is to really let your body relax—and not tense up—during that five-second count. Over time, it trains your nose to increase the volume of air that it's taking in. Some have used this technique to reverse what they call "chronic hyperventilation."

- *Advanced breathing.* As you dig deeper into this area of optimization, you'll find all kinds of breath retention and exhalation exercises, both ancient and new, complex and simple. Wim Hof, whom I referenced earlier, incorporates breathing exercises with cold exposure and has a number of different breathing techniques helping to push all the CO_2 out of the body so that it can stay warm. His breathing techniques require a bit more instruction, but I've found them to be interesting and helpful. Recently, I had the opportunity to see Wim in person, where he shared breathing techniques beyond just simple "nose breathing" in yoga. During this event, I had the most powerful experience following Wim's simple guidance. It was quite the magic moment to feel such euphoria after an exercise like this. If you're eager to try one yourself, there are Wim Hof trainers all over the country that are able to teach the techniques to large groups. While there are very clear benefits to some of these advanced breathing techniques, they require a lot more effort, time, and training, and that means spending more money on your end. Don't try to do advanced breathing exercises on your own for the first time without an instructor.

No matter what technique you choose to experiment with, try to incorporate it into your life as a practice. It's no risk, no cost, and takes little investment of your time—but the benefits are numerous: increased awareness, presence, surrender, and peace. This is something that you can do outside of the meditation time you've carved out. Here's an example: take a moment before a big meeting or conference call and focus on making ten big, steady breaths. Turn off your stereo in your car and focus on your breathing while you drive. Before you eat a meal, sit still and take a few big breaths. As I've mentioned, breathing is one of the only body functions that just naturally happens, but it's also something you can control and use to your advantage. It's much more difficult to modify your heart rate without inputting something physical like running or jumping, but breathing can be *modified* and *improved* by simply implementing breathing techniques once or twice throughout your day.

If it's intimidating to add another practice to your day, then just simply do a breathing exercise whenever it comes to your mind, or whenever you get stressed. Listen to your body. It'll tell you what it needs. In our stress-filled world, oftentimes, you just need to breathe. If you've identified focus, stress, and irritability as issues to try to improve within the framework, there's no reason why you shouldn't be incorporating breathing techniques throughout the day—it's low cost, low effort, and has a high return.

KEY TAKEAWAYS

I've heard hundreds of stories from people who have had transformative experiences with yoga. Like me, they were focused on improving their health and wellness through diet, nutrition, and exercise, but eventually found that mindfulness practice was the missing link. This helped them to improve focus and reduce stress in a world filled with distractions and demands. Mindfulness can get you back to some of life's essentials: breath, awareness, presence, gratitude, and peace.

Get deeper insight into the practice of mindfulness and the benefits of yoga and meditation at www.unstoppablebook.com/chapter16.

CHAPTER 17

LIFE

Fifteen years ago, if you'd told me I'd be writing a book that dealt, in part, with starting a yoga practice and becoming more mindful, I would've said you were crazy. Back then, I wasn't very open to ideas like this, yet following other people's advice regarding nutrition and exercise left me empty, both physically *and* emotionally. It was only through my sheer exhaustion and inability to get the results I wanted that I finally opened myself up to the possibility of alternative practices and methodologies like the ones I've outlined in previous chapters. That's why I feel strongly that in order to become unstoppable, you must open yourself up to possibility, to learning, and to change.

By opening myself up to yoga and the practice of mindfulness, I learned one of the most important concepts of my adult life: the concept of being "present." Presence was something I'd never really thought about before in depth, but, thanks to mindfulness, suddenly I could tell what presence was and what it wasn't. For example, on days that I didn't do yoga, I could pinpoint certain things within myself that I never would've been able to identify before. I could feel a certain distraction—a literal lack of presence—in my mind throughout the workday, which left me feeling disconnected from what was happening. Without yoga, my monkey brain seemed prone to frustration. Worst of all, I could feel myself becoming less understanding with my kids in the evening. My heart just wasn't engaged or present in their matters the way it could be. But when I'd taken the time to do yoga, *to practice being present*, it was entirely different. This was—and continues to be—the undeniable power of presence.

What's great about evolving is that once you've experienced optimization in a certain area of your life, you'll be able to more easily sense when something is "off" in that area down the line. You'll understand your potential more fully, and you'll have ways of getting back on the right track when you go off course, whether that's yoga, meditation, or something else entirely.

In the pages that follow, I will share some more high-level ideas about cultivating mindfulness with yourself and in relationships. Remember, optimization is about making the most of what you have and enjoying life with the form of abundance before you. In relationships, that means enjoying and cultivating the connections you have with partners, children, and friends. By really being present and attentive with those people, and experiencing the fullness of the moment, you'll optimize and maximize your experience of life's richness and beauty.

RELATIONSHIPS WITH PARTNERS

It may seem strange to think about "optimizing" relationships, but in this context, optimization doesn't involve metrics or measurement. Instead, it involves cultivating the connection we have with our partners through mindfulness and being fully present when spending time together. In this context, being "present" can be thought of as *noticing*—noticing yourself and your partner—in order to identify the small ways you can remove the barriers to intimacy that are constructed in modern life. When we notice these things, we can implement practices that prevent the creation and reinforcement of these barriers.

Here's an example: we live in a noisy world these days. It's easy to absentmindedly scroll through your phone while sitting on the couch with a loved one, not really addressing one another, not really *noticing* one another, even though you're sitting in the same room. Even though this can be fine from time to time as a way to relax and unwind, if made into a habit, it can stand in the way of you noticing your partner and cultivating intimacy with them in a meaningful way. That's why I try to leave my phone by the door when I get home. It doesn't mean I always succeed in not being distracted by the day, but it means I've leveraged this practice to give my girlfriend and children the attention they deserve.

Another thing we've built into our routine?

Dedicated one-on-one time with my girlfriend. That means implementing a weekly date night or seasonal weekend away with one another. Remember, the purpose of routine is to free you up to be more present. If you both know that you're going to have a date night every other Friday, for example, then that eliminates the potential stress of not knowing when you're going to get one-on-one time with your partner. If there's something serious that you know you need to talk to him or her about, or if you just feel like you need some one-on-one time with someone who is special to you, then knowing you've got a weekly date night planned can alleviate stress and keep your heart and mind in a state of equanimity. If you're in a romantic relationship, something else that I recommend doing is committing to getting away every three to six months for a weekend. Turn your phones and electronics off when you get where you're going—this time is for you. It doesn't have to be fancy, either: go camping, or to a nearby city and rent out an Airbnb. You'll be surprised how much you grow as a couple when this kind of intention is at play and there's nothing to distract you.

Another thing that I build into my routine (and this one's a little bit out there) is negative visualization. Whenever I start to get negative, reactive, or self-absorbed, I remind myself that nothing is permanent in life. This kind of negative visualization helps me to grow in appreciation for what I have in the present, without irrational passion or attachment. This is an aspect of stoicism, a life philosophy where I've found some inspiration. Whenever I am with my family or friends, or even working on a project or pursuing an idea I'm excited about, I remind myself that I'm not always going to be here. This helps me to ground myself and have an appreciation and gratitude for that moment in time.

HAVING AND RAISING KIDS

Everyone always says that your life changes when you have kids. That's certainly true to some extent, but I think that one reason why parents say this is because they don't understand how to integrate parenting into how they used to live. And so, their previous way of "living" and their new lives as parents become compartmentalized. Thinking that all the "fun" they used to have as a couple is now over because kids are in the picture can cause significant grief and bitterness within a relationship, and can even cause disdain for your own children.

Even though my girlfriend and I have children, we still do all the things we used to do. We've tried not to change what we're doing or want to do, and instead, we just integrate the kids more. The biggest change was that we increased our prioritization of experiences for the whole family. When our daughter was two weeks old, we started taking her out to dinner with us. Show your children that you're incorporating them into the things that you love and the traditions that you have established. There's no need to make them feel as if they're separate from your relationship with your partner. In fact, this could actually be quite confusing psychologically for them. Take them on your date nights and your weekend getaways and your trips—just not always. Take them on a walk around the city. Take them on a hike. Though it's inevitable that your life will change in some ways when you have kids, for practical purposes, it doesn't have to change *drastically*. It's about prioritization, and the more you can focus on experiences over accumulating things, something my girlfriend has helped me to understand, the easier this is.

Just like your relationship with your partner, the goal with your children is to experience genuine connection with them every single day. We try to get them outside and away from electronics. Maybe that means playing board games, making arts and crafts, building something new and interesting, or competing in a sport outside. If we do watch a movie or a show, it's something that we all try to do together. We see no need for each of our kids to be binge-watching something different in separate rooms. If we're going to do something that involves electronics, we want to use it as an opportunity for genuine connection or learning, or both—to laugh together, or get absorbed in a story together, or whatever it may be.

OTHER AREAS OF EXPERIMENTATION TO OPTIMIZE YOUR HEART AND MIND

Most people go to bed focusing on what went wrong with their day. It might be that dreaded feeling that they didn't get things done and are overwhelmed with how much more there still is to do. It might be the email they received that caused anxiety to build up within them. It might be criticism from their boss, or a conflict with their spouse. It could be something they saw on the internet, or drama in the news. Whatever the source, the great curse of the human brain is that it tends to focus on what's *wrong* in life. It takes hard work to retrain your mind to focus on what's right, and to let gratitude and love define the moments of your day. Here are some of the simple things that you can do in your life to create more space for positivity and let go of the things that are holding you back:

- *Cut out television, social media, and news, especially in the evenings.* I used to be a person who had CNN on at all times throughout the workday. I liked having noise in the background. I liked being in touch with what was going on in the world, or so I thought. The reality, however, is that the news actually is *not* a good representation of what's going on, just a biased and negative set of things shared with you to cause fear or moral outrage. The idea isn't to inform—it's to get you addicted, and boost their ratings in the process.
- Back when I was watching CNN every day, one week the live stream stopped working with my internet connection at the office. The interruption in my routine was a catalyst for me to wonder, "What would my day be like without the endless news cycle as soundtrack?" I decided to answer this question, testing my exposure to the news, and measuring how I felt in response. I did this for about a week. The next week I turned the news back on again. What I realized is that I was much less focused the following morning whenever I had the news on the previous day. My brain was more reactive and more difficult to tame. I decided to commit to giving up the news during the day and even eventually stopped watching it at night. It helped me to focus more on the task at hand during the day and be more connected to my family at night. And, as far as being informed, the truth was that, if anything big happened in the news, I could spend ten to fifteen

minutes online in the evening educating myself on the happenings of the day. If anything major happened, like a terrorist attack or natural disaster, I'd probably hear about it from a friend or family member via call or text. Never in the history of the world have human beings had immediate access to national and global news via around-the-clock coverage and social media—and this accessibility isn't always a good thing. Most of the news has no personal effect on you, other than implanting negativity into your brain.

- *Limit social media.* I recognize that some people need social media for work and that others put it to good use staying connected to long-distance family and friends, but social media has to be carefully monitored and managed. Social media has been linked to anxiety, irrational comparisons, judgment, and depression. Strict boundaries need to be drawn. When I had social media apps on my phone, I found that in my spare time or during moments in the day when I was waiting for something, I'd just automatically start pulling up the different apps on my phone to kill the time. Rather than daydreaming, thinking, being in the moment, or breathing, I would trigger my monkey brain while scrolling through different social feeds. Once I removed these apps, there was much more creative space, problem-solving time, deep-thought time, and most importantly, *presence.* It took almost no effort, just commitment—and the results were huge. At that time, I removed all social media apps from my phone. Now I only get on social media occasionally on my computer if it's work-related. If you have to have it, just know that these apps are designed by intelligent people and marketers whose primary goal is to get your brain addicted to using their product. Think about how dangerous that is to the high-functioning power of your brain. When we're not busy wasting time, there's an opportunity to let our minds roam freely—this is why some of the best ideas come to your mind while you're in the shower or in a physical environment that's unlike the majority of your day. Create more freedom for your mind, and imagine what you can dream up and do.

• *Consider another way to accomplish the tasks you don't love to do.* Unless you've got the financial freedom to pay for things to be done that you don't enjoy doing, recognize that each of us will have to complete tasks that aren't enjoyable. But most have never even considered the question, "Is there another way to accomplish this task so that I don't have to do it?" Most just think they're stuck having to do a wide range of things that they don't want to do, when the reality is that life's a bit more malleable than that. Working with your partner to understand how you can accomplish household and related tasks based on preference or familiarity can be helpful, as long as you're sharing the burden. Push to find out how certain tasks, for example, cleaning the house, can be shared, or perhaps eliminated altogether, by hiring someone who can help. Make time to utilize your own talents and the things in life that you enjoy. You'll feel happier, more fulfilled, and have more energy.

- *Remove negative and stressful people from your life.* So many people are stuck in toxic relationships and friendships, or are constantly around those who suck the energy right out of them. Though it's impossible to remove everyone from your life whom you don't enjoy being around, you can create boundaries in relationships in every area of your life to protect yourself, and your energy. Don't take the bait from toxic people. Don't let yourself get pulled into the pointlessness of gossip or drama. Find people that make your life better.

- *Read, learn, and rejuvenate your mind.* When considering optimization, the tendency is to view this in the context of all the things that you have to do, or give, throughout the day. Though this is true in some ways, optimization is also about finding ways to get your energy back, via sleep and/or nutrition. You can't give your energy all day long and never let yourself rest or rejuvenate on a mental and emotional level. Use the extra time and space you have made for yourself (through cutting out the unnecessary distractions I discussed) to perhaps read a good book or listen to an inspiring talk. You could even spend time learning about any of the ideas in this book! Replace the background sounds of television and news with TED Talks and audio books. Like mindfulness, reading and learning are areas in which you can relax and rejuvenate and, at the same time, sharpen your mind and develop perspective.

Learning is at the heart of your journey. The goal of this chapter is to get you to think about areas you might not typically even consider as something that could be optimized. Expand the mind to the possibilities that are out there—the possibilities that can really bring lasting improvement to your life. Open yourself up to learning in those areas.

I would never have found testing and optimization in business if it weren't for my desire to learn, and I would have never applied this framework to my life if it weren't for my desire to learn about health and wellness. One of the gifts I was given as a child was not only going to a progressive school, where we were taught how to learn and problem solve, but because of my learning disability, I truly learned how to understand my mind, and learn in a way that worked for me. Adapt the framework to your unique learning style and see where your learning takes you.

For more resources and information about optimizing relationships, go to www.unstoppablebook.com/chapter17.

CONCLUSION

I've often said to many friends and family members that if I ever had six-pack abs, I wouldn't even own a shirt. That might sound weird to some of you, but for anyone who has ever struggled with their weight or self-image, you probably get it. I've worked so hard to get my weight down over the years. I've followed rigid formulas. I've stuck to schedules. I've disciplined myself in ridiculous ways. No matter what I've done, or how religious I've been, shame, frustration, and self-judgment have consistently resurfaced in my life. If I ever had six-pack abs, I think I'd be so proud that I would want to relish that success every moment of every day. It has been a long, difficult journey.

Truthfully, even in implementing the Unstoppable Lifestyle over the last several years, I'm still hard on myself when I look in the mirror or put on a pair of pants. I'm not here to sugarcoat things or act as if I'm perfect. I'm still experimenting. I'm still learning. I'm still evolving. In fact, I've accepted that I might always struggle with my weight and self-image. But I will say this: I do feel better than I've ever felt in my life. Though I don't have six-pack abs, I'm not constantly hungry, and I no longer feel fat. I feel free.

When I first started doing yoga, I had a certain envy for the men who would take their shirts off during class. It was hard for me to ever imagine doing such a thing, even though most of those who were taking off their shirts didn't have six-pack abs. But my body had always been the source of shame and frustration. Taking my shirt off seemed incomprehensible. But the more I followed the framework I've outlined in this book, what I now call the Unstoppable Lifestyle, the better I felt. And the more I tried to apply the principles of yoga to the rest of my life—like nonjudgment, presence, breath, and acceptance—the more confident I became. I finally began to accept my body and even *like* my body. As yogis will sometimes say, "Meet your body where it is today." That's what I began to do.

And then one day in yoga class, something crazy happened: without even thinking about it, I took off my shirt.

Although I'd never done that before, it felt natural. It felt good. It felt right. For such a long time, I'd been frustrated with my body, and, on my worst days, even felt cursed to have the body I had. But that day in yoga—and every day since—I've wanted to celebrate my body for the gift that it is, even if I don't have six-pack abs.

There's another yogi saying I love: "The teacher in me recognizes the teacher in all of you." For me, this saying is a reminder that even those of us who've come a long way still have much to learn, and vice versa. The commonality is that we're all on our own journey. No one is better than the other. If nothing else, this encapsulates the gentleness with which we must all address all areas of improvement within our lives.

The most important lesson I've learned in my own journey is that my body—and *your* body—is worth celebrating. No matter where you're at on your journey, your body should be viewed as a gift, even if it's not "perfect." Because regardless of how we look and how healthy we feel, our bodies have the power to guide us in the right direction. Often, the hardest thing is just learning to listen to it.

So, keep going. Keep evolving. And to put my own twist on that yogi saying, the learner in me recognizes the learner in you.

ABOUT THE AUTHOR

DAVID HAUSER is a serial entrepreneur who launched several companies before he began high school. David spent his youth working more than one hundred hours a week, until he realized the toll it was taking on his mind, body, and life. After failing to see results from conventional wisdom, he decided to do what he does best: innovate. His unique journey to wellness has helped him realize his life's purpose of empowering others to optimize their own lives by reclaiming their health. As David continues to evolve, he receives tremendous support from his partner, Dawn, and their three inspiring children.